THE OFFICIAL
JOHN WAYNE
HANDY BOOK FOR MEN

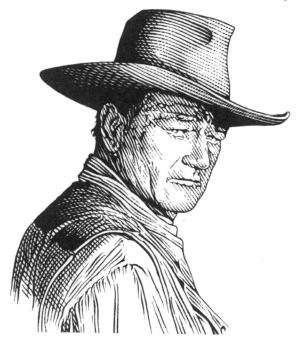

Fountaindale Public Library
Bolingbrook, IL
(630) 759-2102

JAMES ELLIS

ILLUSTRATIONS BY T.M. DETWILER
COVER ILLUSTRATION BY RICHARD PHIPPS/ILLUSTRATIONWEB.COM

"GODDAMN, I'M THE STUFF MEN ARE MADE OF!"

—JOHN WAYNE

EING A MAN MEANS different things to different people. For some, masculinity is tied to the distant past, when man was responsible for building a fire no matter the weather, foraging for food no matter the season and fighting off danger no matter its form. For others, a man's defining characteristic is his ability to accept responsibility for his actions. But these are strange times and ideas about what makes a man have become hazy, indistinct and are often in dispute.

Luckily, we have an unforgettable role model to cut through the confusion and show us what real masculinity, and the rugged individuality that defines it, looks like— John Wayne. Duke, idolized as the epitome of manliness for generations, could drive cattle in the morning, chop down a tree in the afternoon, prepare a romantic dinner for his lady before the sun went down and call it just another average day.

Inspired by John Wayne's classic values of grit, honor and loyalty, not to mention his all-around aptitude in all things badass, this book has instructions and advice for performing more than 100 skills every man should know.

You may not be John Wayne by the time you turn the last page—but you'll be the next best thing, and that ain't bad.

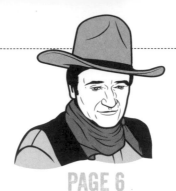

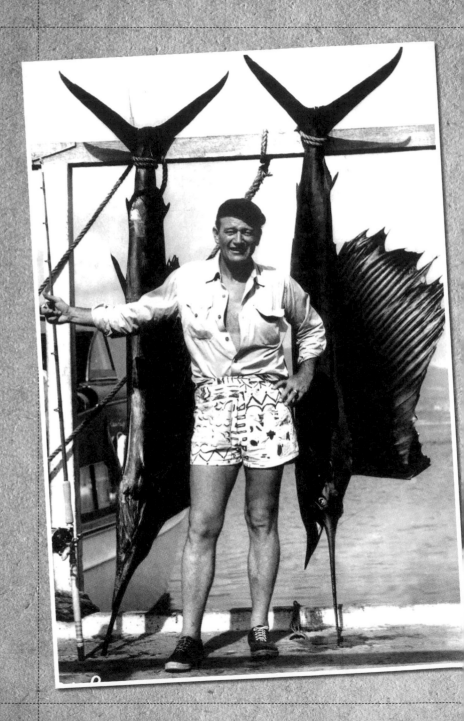

THE GREAT OUTDOORS

HANDLE YOURSELF WISELY IN AMERICA'S BEAUTIFUL BUT DEADLY LANDSCAPES

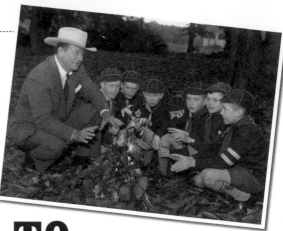

Duke warms up by a campfire with some Scouts during a visit to Ottershaw, U.K., 1960.

HOW TO BUILD A FIRE

O ABILITY separates the competent individualist from the pretenders better than starting a fire in the wilderness. Anyone can conjure flames with a lighter or matches (which are still wise to carry while outdoors), but you're better than that. Using nothing but your wits, grit and what Mother Nature provides, you can build a bonfire signalling your superiority over the elements—provided you follow the advice below.

1. *SET YOUR SITE*
From start to finish, it may take more than an hour to conjure flames from the wilderness, so try not to begin during the last few minutes of daylight. You want someplace dry and sheltered from the wind, which can snuff out your embers before they grow into something capable of warming you up. Also avoid spots with dry grass or leaves—you do not want a forest fire. Clear all flammables in a 10-foot radius to be safe.

2. *GET TINDER*
Start looking for any dry, lightweight material that will easily ignite (think twigs, dry grass or wood shavings).

You'll also need to find kindling, such as dry branches you might find at the base of a tree, that will feed your small flame without being so heavy as to smother them. Finally, you'll want to gather fuel, larger pieces of wood to feed your fire and keep you warm throughout the night.

3. *PILE IT UP*

Prop up pieces of your kindling against a large log or part of a downed, dead tree provided neither is surrounded by other flammable flora and place the tinder in the space between the kindling and whatever it's leaning against. Once you've ignited the tinder, the lean-to protects the fragile flame from wind and allows it to set the larger kindling on fire.

4. *LET THERE BE LIGHT*

Assuming you aren't carrying a lighter or matches, you have several options when in the wild, but the simplest one relies on friction. Find a dry, sturdy stick about 3 feet in length and sharpen one end to a point with a knife or sharp rock. Then procure another dry, flat piece of wood that will act as your fireboard. Use your knife to make a small notch in the flat board, then take the sharpened stick and place it perpendicular to the fireboard, with the sharp end pressing down in the notch. Place the palms of your hands on either side of the stick and roll it back and forth between them rapidly while pressing down at the same time. After a considerable amount of effort, you should turn the sharp end of the stick into a glowing ember.

5. *BLOW THEM AWAY*

This hot ember is now your life. Love it. Protect it. Carefully bring it to your pile of tinder until it (hopefully) ignites. Now gently blow on your tiny flame to feed it oxygen (but not enough to snuff it out). Soon, you should have a serviceable fire you can feed fuel as needed. That warmth you feel? It isn't just from the flame—it's also from the satisfaction that comes from triumphing over nature.

HOW TO BUILD A SHELTER

HE DAY MAY COME when you find yourself stranded in the wilderness, far away from the comforts afforded by four solid walls and a roof over your head. Fortunately for you, the following information ensures you'll never be caught out in the cold again by guiding you through the basics of constructing a simple shelter with nothing but pure determination.

1. *GET THE LAY OF THE LAND*
The most important decision you have to make when constructing your shelter is its eventual location. Common sense will serve you well here—pick someplace where the ground is as dry as possible, and avoid selecting a spot directly underneath a cliff or dead tree where you are in danger of getting hit by falling debris. Also, don't build your shelter in a ravine or valley if it can be helped, or you run the risk of getting swept up in a flash flood if a sudden downpour spoils your plans.

2. *GET FRAMED*
Look around for a straight, sturdy branch a few feet longer than you are tall, as well as at least six other shorter branches (about 4 or 5 feet in length) that are also reasonably straight and free from deformity. Prop two of the shorter sticks into the shape of an "A," lashing them together with a belt, shoelaces

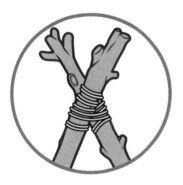

or any natural twine, grass or soft branches that may be at hand (if the ground is soft enough, you could also simply jam the sticks into the soil to keep them in the desired "A" shape). Now place one end of the longer stick on the top of this "A," (or for extra durability, tie it to the top of the "A") and rest the other end on the ground. Next, lean your other shorter branches against both sides of the longer branch to construct the frame of your shelter and tie together.

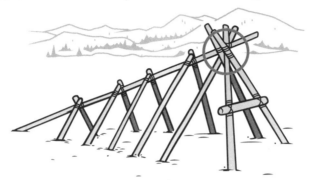

3. *COVER UP*
To insulate your shelter as much as possible, gather smaller branches and place them against the frame. Next, take any nearby debris (leaves, smaller branches, etc.) and pile it on to those branches. You now have a temporary shelter against the elements that will help keep you alive as you plan your way back to safety.

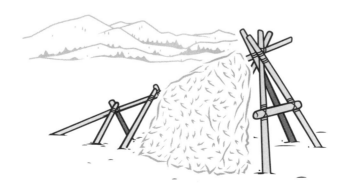

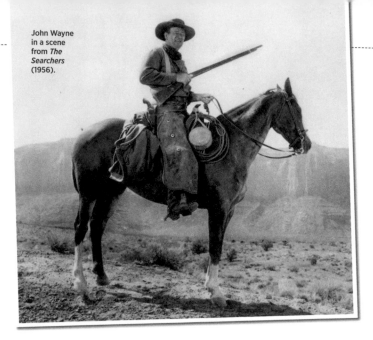

John Wayne in a scene from *The Searchers* (1956).

HOW TO FOLLOW A TRACK

 EING A RUGGED and independent individual in a world full of less-capable folks comes with responsibility. Just as Duke wouldn't abandon a town of peaceful settlers to fend for themselves against merciless outlaws or leave a wagon train in need of his guidance, neither should you callously turn your back on those who need your help. A time may come when you have to help find a lost friend (or stranger) in the woods before danger locates that person first. Here's how to track 'em down.

1. *KEEP YOUR EYES OPEN*
Go to the last known place the missing was spotted and study your surroundings. You want to zero in on anomalies in the environment that are clearly man made. Search for signs like trampled grass, footprints, torn

spider webs and tracked mud. You won't see these tracks if you're directly on top of them, so try to look at the scene from multiple angles.

2. *USE YOUR HEAD*

Once you've found a clue, you're going to want to inspect it through sideheading. This means getting low to the ground and turning your head sideways to get a different perspective. This will allow you to see shadows better, giving you a more accurate impression of where tracks are going. Pay attention to the footprint itself. If one is deeper than the other, the target may be favoring one of their legs. If the footsteps are deeper and closer together they were probably walking, whereas prints that are farther apart indicate running.

3. *KEEP USING YOUR HEAD*

You also should use common sense when tracking down the lost. Is there a nearby trail or paved path in the area? Chances are any practical person stumbling upon a trail would follow it rather than continue to wander in the woods. If you have a map of the area, draw a circle that spans three miles in each direction from the lost person's last known position, as nearly half of lost hikers can be found within that area. Start your search there and it may be over sooner than you expect.

4. *NEVER GIVE UP*

Just because you lost the trail doesn't mean you should call it quits. Try to clear your mind of frustration and focus on the task at hand. Getting focused on your failures can cloud your judgement and discourage you from picking up newer, more important clues. No one disappears into thin air—they will always leave behind some trace. That said, if you can't find who you're looking for alone, there can be strength in numbers, even for the rugged individualist. Get a posse together and fan out, expanding your search by expanding the size of your group.

HOW TO HANG FOOD FROM A TREE

NYONE WHO KNOWS anything about camping will bring with them plenty of vittles and provisions to keep their bellies full on the trip. Unfortunately, the same foodstuff we like to chow down on around the fire also attracts all sorts of animals that have evolved to track down sources of sustenance no matter the cost. To avoid having a close encounter with a rummaging intruder that leaves you stranded without rations or mauled in your sleep, follow the steps below to keep your supplies safe.

1. *ASSEMBLE YOUR GEAR*
Get together anything that could attract an animal to your camp such as uneaten food, trash, toothpaste and even sunblock. Place these items in a light, nylon bag that can be easily hung. Grab a long rope, preferably 100 feet, a carabiner (a specialized metal loop you can buy at any camping supply store) and a heavy rock. Don't have a carabiner handy? Check page 66 for knots that'll effectively solve that problem.

2. *LOOK FOR TALL TREES*
Now it's time to figure out where you're going to place your food. Get at least 200 feet away from your camp just in case this doesn't work. Once you're far away, start looking for a pair of trees that are at least 15 feet tall and 20 feet apart. Make sure their branches are heavy enough to support your bag.

3. *HANG YOUR ROPE*

Next, tie one end of your rope to your rock and the other end to the first tree's trunk. Now throw the rock up over one of that tree's branches. Once that's accomplished, throw the rock over a branch of equal height on the second tree. Leave a decent amount of slack between the two branches.

4. *HANG YOUR BAG*

Go to the center of the two trees and tie a loop in the slack section of rope there. Take your carabiner and use it to attach your bag to this loop. Make sure the bag isn't near any trees, that way a bear can't easily climb to it.

5. *HOIST YOUR BAG*

Pull on the rope to hoist up the bag and tie the free end to the second tree trunk. This will secure the bag and ensure it does not fall later on.

BEAR NECESSITIES

Hanging food from a tree is a vital step in making sure your campsite doesn't become a food court for bears, but far from the only one. In general, bears don't enjoy loud noises but love to investigate any area from which delicious (or even just pungent) smells emit, so plan accordingly. That might mean forgoing frying up a rasher of bacon in the morning if you know you're hiking through bear country or making sure you wear something that generates noise throughout your trek, such as a bear bell. And it's not only the food you put into you that can attract bears but also the waste you expel. Make sure you "do your business" a ways away from camp (about 100 yards) to help cut down on the chances of a bear tracking you down.

HOW TO ALWAYS FIND TRUE NORTH

 IVING LIFE to the fullest means losing your way every now and again. After all, sticking to the script and staying inside the boundaries of a map means missing out on all of the adventures out there waiting for you. When it's time for you to get back on track, remember the tips below to reliably find north so you can keep on keepin' on.

1. *STICK WITH IT*

If the sun is high in the sky, find a stick a couple of feet in length and stick it straight into the ground. Place a rock or some other object that will stay put at the end of the shadow the stick casts. Wait about 15 minutes and use another object to mark the end of the shadow. Stand with your back to the stick, the front of your left toe touching the first object and the front of your right toe touching the second. Congratulations. You're now facing true north.

2. *NEEDLEPOINT*

If you happen to have a metal needle on you (maybe you were traveling with a sewing kit or, marginally more likely, a first-aid kit), and a puddle of water nearby, this method of getting your bearings is fairly simple. In truth, you don't necessarily need something labeled "needle" in bold letters—a bent paper clip or stripped piece of wire could also do in a pinch. Take a scrap of wool or silk (hopefully you have some clothing you can rip) and rub it from end-to-end on your needle about 100 times to magnetize it. Place the needle on a leaf or something else that is buoyant and place that on the water's surface. The needle should point to either true north or true south—there's no way to tell which end points to which, so look for the sun (if it is out) which always rises in the east and sets in the west. You should be able to orient yourself north using both the sun and the needle.

3. *STARRY NIGHT*

A clear night with the stars visible is a dream come true to anyone looking for north. If you're north of the equator (and you really should know that without any special skills), look for the Big Dipper. You can usually find it about a third of the way up from the horizon. The bright star on the top right corner of the cradle part of the Big Dipper is the North Star, which shows the way north. If you're Down Under (or in New Zealand or anywhere else in the Southern Hemisphere), find the constellation known as the Southern Cross (start by spotting the two bright stars near it known as The Pointers) and then extend the axis of the Cross in your mind's eye toward the horizon. That's true south, which orients you just as well true north does.

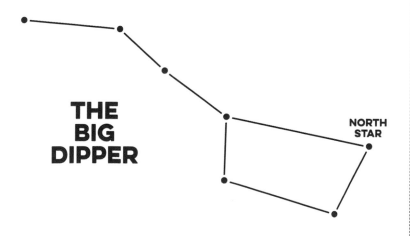

THE BIG DIPPER

NORTH STAR

HOW TO RIDE A HORSE

 VERYONE HAS DREAMS about riding as tall in the saddle as John Wayne, but it takes a mixture of guts, intuition and skill to climb on the back of an animal weighing more than 1,000 pounds and tell it where to go. These basics of horsemanship will set you on the path to the rodeo.

1. *START HORSE WHISPERING*
Before you can mount your horse, you should do a small amount of prep work. First, make sure the horse is calm; an anxious horse will fidget and make mounting difficult.

2. *MOUNT UP!*
Next, positioning yourself on the left side of the horse, firmly grab the reins with your left hand. While the reason for this lies in tradition and not science, chances are your horse has been broken in by riders mounting from the left and a beginner shouldn't try to buck tradition...unless he enjoys getting bucked from a horse. Continue to hold on to the horse's reins as you place your left foot in the stirrup. Once your foot is secure, lift your body weight up using the stirrup and throw your right leg over the horse. Place yourself firmly on the horse as you position your right foot in its stirrup. Make sure to keep your back straight and your knees turned inward. Don't squeeze the horse tightly, but be firm—like a good parent, you're never cruel but you need to establish who is in charge.

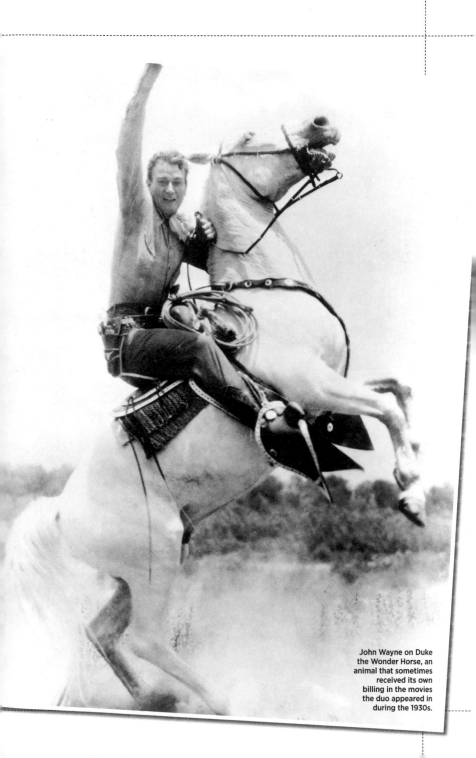

John Wayne on Duke the Wonder Horse, an animal that sometimes received its own billing in the movies the duo appeared in during the 1930s.

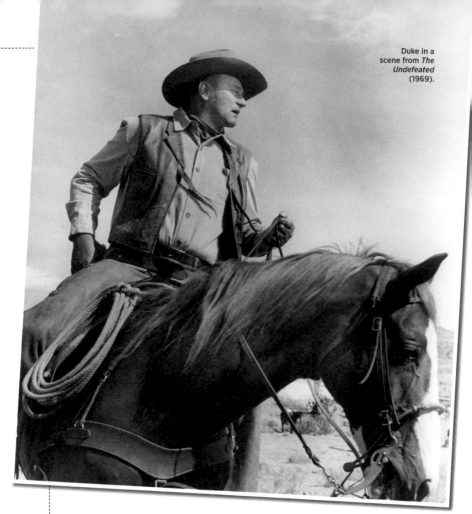

3. *GRAB THE REINS*

Place the reins in both of your hands in the proper fashion. Let the reins rest on the inside of your middle three fingers. Form a loose fist so the reins drape over your thumb and pinky finger. Turn your fists so your thumbs point up and slightly toward each other.

4. *GET MOVING*

Your horse will start walking forward when you give it a gentle squeeze with your knees. Most horses are trained to walk forward when given this subtle command.

Get used to the horse's rhythm as it walks, being careful not to pull the reins in the opposite direction of its bobbing head.

5. *KEEP HER STEADY*
Steering your horse is relatively easy to figure out. Reins are the basis of control; lightly pulling on one will typically make the horse move in that direction. Pushing your knees lightly into a horse's side will also influence it to move in the opposite direction. For example: Steering left can be accomplished both by pulling on the left rein or by applying pressure with your right knee.

6. *HOT TO TROT*
Once you're moving in the right direction you can give your steed a quick, hard squeeze with your legs to set the horse in a trot. Placing your weight in the balls of your feet will make trotting more comfortable.

7. *GIDDYUP*
Loosening the reins slightly and leaning forward will increase the horse's speed. This is why keeping your back straight is so important, because even a casual lean could send your horse galloping forward. Leaning completely forward will cause the horse to break into a full run, while placing your weight at the back of the saddle and tightening the reins will slow it down. Make sure never to pull too hard on the horse, as this will jerk its head backward and irritate it.

8. *GETTING OFF*
Once you're finished with your ride, bring the horse to a halt and take both feet from the stirrups. Hold the reins in your left hand and the pommel of the saddle in the other. Then smoothly lean forward, lift up your right leg and swing it over your mount's rear to land beside your trusty steed.

HOW TO
MAKE A SNARE

 N A SURVIVAL SITUATION, food is never going to be the first thing on your list of necessities. Finding shelter and water should be your first concerns, as the elements and thirst will prove intolerable long before the rumbling in your stomach becomes debilitating. But, a man's gotta eat at some point, and a simple wire snare can be one of the most useful tools for trapping small game, whether you're stranded or just out to prove you're a wilderness master.

When stranded in the wild, both time and energy conservation are of the utmost importance. Even the most skilled tracker and hunter will eventually tire, especially if their food supply is already limited. A snare, once made, is set and left, allowing you to rest, build a fire, repair your shelter or try to get rescued while your snare does the hard work of acquiring small game for you to survive on.

1. *WHAT YOU NEED*

A snare consists of two very simple parts: a wire element and a fastener element. If you're the kind of always-prepared person who keeps an emergency kit around, for less than $10 you can find everything you need to have several traps stored away in case of a survival situation. The ideal materials are picture wire and small metal fasteners called cable ferrules to make up the snare itself. In a pinch, wire from headphones, electronics, spiral notebooks or even bras can be used just as well. If all else fails, any rope or cordage available will do. For the fastener, the only requirement is that the cord be able to fit twice through the fastener to create a loop.

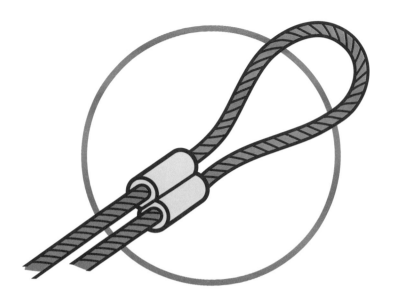

2. *FASHION YOUR NOOSE*

With a multi-tool or wire cutters, trim a piece of wire between 24" and 36". Loop one end through your fastener and bend it back around, creating a loop about the diameter of a pencil.

3. *CRIMP IT AND CLOSE IT*

Use your wire cutters to crimp down your fastener, holding the wire in place. Don't use too much force and risk cutting through the fastener. Wrap the remaining part of the short end of the wire around the long end to close the first end of your noose. Now, pass the other end of your wire through the loop, creating the circle into which your prey will eventually run (pictured).

4. *REPEAT*

Bend, fasten and close the end of your wire as above to create a second loop.

5. *LAY YOUR NOOSE*

Using paracord, rope, string, shoelaces or whatever is available, tie the free end of the snare to a sturdy branch near a well-traveled game path—you can tell one by the presence of tracks and droppings—and place the noose low to the ground, lightly resting on another tree branch or stick that you've propped up for this purpose. As the animal passes through the snare, its forward movement will tighten the circle, effectively trapping it.

6. *KEEP AN EYE OUT*

Check your traps covertly every 4–6 hours, or even a bit more often if you're able. More often than not this style of snare simply traps rather than kills the animal, making it possible for your dinner to wriggle or chew its way out. It would also be a shame if another predator came along and took advantage of all your hard work.

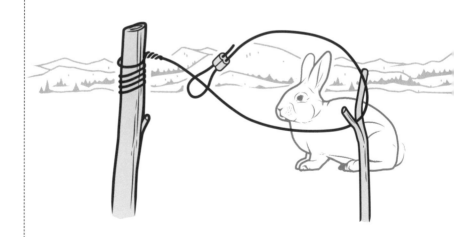

HOW TO SKIN YOUR GAME

Once you've caught your dinner, you still have a few chores to take care of before that bunny can make its way into your belly. The most gruesome task ahead of you is skinning and gutting the animal, but while messy, this doesn't have to be a big production.

1. Take a sharp knife or object and make a cut on the underside of the animal where the tail meets the body, creating a loose flap of skin.

2. Grab the animal by its hind legs and pin that loose flap of skin to the ground with your foot, so you can skin the animal from feet to head by pulling upward.

3. Now that you have your animal skinned, carefully cut open the underside of the animal without piercing the stomach or bladder (which can ruin the meat). Remove the organs so there is a hollow cavity left, and congratulate yourself for field dressing your prey.

HOW TO CHOP DOWN A TREE WITH AN AX

REES ARE ONE of nature's greatest gifts, providing us with shade, beauty and oxygen. But sometimes, they gotta go. There are likely plenty of services in your area that'll solve the problem, but if you'd prefer to fell a tree on your own, read below to find out how to do it efficiently and safely.

1. *EXAMINE YOUR WORK SPACE*
Before you make a single mark on that tree, you first need to study it and make sure you can safely cut it down. If the tree leans in one particular direction, that's where it will fall, so make sure your house, car, children, John Wayne movie collection, etc. aren't in its path. You can use the ax method to determine the distance of clear space you'll need to make space for the tree once it topples. Hold your ax handle straight up and down at arm's length, make like Rooster Cogburn and look at it with one eye, then take steps either toward or away from the tree until the top of the ax is aligned with the treetop and the bottom is aligned with the base. Your feet

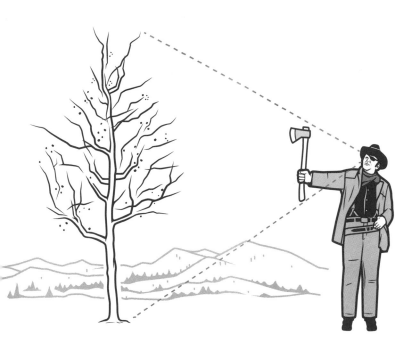

are roughly where the tree will extend to once it falls, but given that this is just an estimate, you'll still want to allow for some extra room beyond where you're standing. Also look up to make sure there aren't large, dead branches supported by other limbs lurking above, ready to drop on your head during the felling process. If there are you'll want to clear those first using your hands, a saw and a ladder or harness system.

2. *MAKE YOUR MARK*

Once you've determined you can go ahead and take down this tree, take your ax and start cutting near the base of the tree facing the direction you want the tree to fall. You should be cutting downward at an angle—not straight on—until you chop through about a third of the tree's diameter.

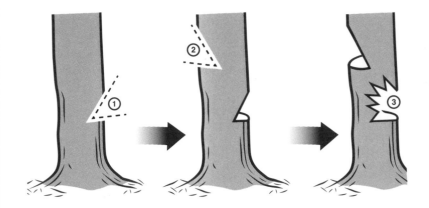

3. *SWITCH SIDES*

Go to the other side of the tree and start a new cut
on the back side of the trunk, a foot or so higher than
your original cut on the front. The goal is to create a
wedge on either side of the tree, with a pillar of wood
remaining in the middle acting as a hinge. Cut about
half way through the diameter of the tree, and then
return to the side of the tree where you made your
original cut.

4. *TIMBER!*

Continue chopping on your original cut, but this time
with an upward angle toward the wedge on the other
side. Pay careful attention here—the tree is ready to
fall, and it can happen more swiftly and quietly than
cartoons would have you believe. Once the tree begins
to fall, run like hell toward the opposite direction. Then
pat yourself on the back for accomplishing a task Duke
would be proud of.

DOES THAT TREE HAVE TO GO?

Now that you know everything there is to know about chopping down a tree, it may behoove you to take a step back and figure out when you should deploy your new skill. When does a tree need to be chopped down? The short answer is if it looks at risk of falling on its own in a way that could cause a lot of damage. If you suspect that oak in your front yard is a potential insurance premium hike waiting to happen, there are a couple of steps you can take to help determine how sick it is.

If the tree is heavily leaning to one side or the other, that's a potential sign all is not well. If the branches of the tree look "loose" in general, as if they aren't connected in a sturdy manner to the trunk, that's another possible indicator of decay. Yet another way to assess the health of the tree is to do a little on-hands investigation. Scratch a small portion of bark off the tree and take a look at the wood underneath. Is it a vibrant green? Great, your tree should be around for the long haul. If the wood is black, however, start sharpening that ax. And if you're married, ask your wife. Always ask your wife.

HOW TO CHOP FIREWOOD

 EW ACTIONS SCREAM "I'm a self-sufficient, rough-n-tough SOB" like chopping firewood with an ax. This time-honored tradition depends on having access to a suitable source of stuff to chop, either harvested from felled trees or, perhaps more realistically, purchased from a trusted local merchant. Once you have the required wood, these instructions will tell you how to get it down to size for you and the whole family to enjoy come winter.

1. *COLLECT YOUR MATERIAL*
To get started, find yourself an ax, goggles and a chopping block. The goggles will keep your peepers safe from bits of wood sent flying by your mighty swings. Your chopping block should be a large, thick piece of unsplit wood (such as a large stump) that is cut parallel on both sides. The purpose of this chopping block is to prevent your ax from hitting the ground if you miss your target (which, of course, you never will), and also saves your back some pain by elevating the target so you don't have to stoop down so low as you chop.

2. *CHOOSE AND POSITION*
Now that you're set up, you need to choose your wood. Find a straight-grained log without knots, and a horizontal surface at each end. The length of wood is up to you, but 14–18 inches is the common length. Position it at the center of your chopping block, with the horizontal surface facing up. If your log has knots, however, make sure to stand it up on the end with the knots (if possible) because wood fibers can cross and get jumbled around these imperfections, leaving an unclean split.

3. *GET CHOPPING*

Now go to town with that ax. Stand with your feet shoulder-width apart and your knees bent. Grab the handle at the base of the blade with your dominant hand and the end of the handle with your other hand. Bring the ax over your head then swing it down, letting gravity and the weight of the ax do most of the work. Keep your focus on the center until your ax has struck the wood. If your log is thick, you might have to strike it a few more times before it fully splits.

4. *STACK AND SIT*

Now that your firewood is chopped, you need to stack it neatly and let it sit. To have the best firewood, you should let it sit for about a year. Having it sit will dehydrate the wood's fiber cells down to about 20 percent. This will make sure your wood burns efficiently, meaning it won't need much attention in order for it to stay lit. You don't need to cover your wood for the entire year either. Instead, cover it a few weeks prior to when you plan on having your fire. Good things take time, so make sure you give your firewood all the time it needs.

HOW TO USE YOUR FIREPLACE

Sure, building a fire in your fireplace might seem as simple as stacking up the firewood and lighting a match. But if you want to make the kind of fire that looks like it should have an entire television channel dedicated to it, you need to take the time to get things started the right way. Place two pieces of firewood so they lay parallel to the back of the fireplace and are six inches apart from each other. Then pile the kindling between these two pieces of wood. Next take an additional two pieces of wood and place them on top of the first two pieces but running perpendicular to the back of the fireplace. After stacking 4-6 logs in this manner, stuff some lint from your dyer in near the lowest level of kindling and light'er up!

HOW TO CLIMB A MOUNTAIN

OST PEOPLE talk about "climbing mountains" as part of a clunky metaphor for surmounting an incredible challenge. One way to test your bonafides as a person who accomplishes the unthinkable is to literally scale a mountain, a task that will require you to summon every scrap of strength, resilience and courage at your disposal. People, even experienced and prepared ones, can die in the attempt, so this isn't for the faint of heart. If you're serious about making the climb, gird yourself for months of training with climbers who know what they're doing. In the meantime, read on to discover some basic survival techniques that will provide a good start to your mountain climbing education.

1. *LISTEN AND LEARN*

Before you grab any climbing gear, you're going to want to hit the books first. No mountain is alike, and they all present their own set of unique challenges. Factors such as weather and height can make all the difference in your ability to complete a climb. Try and find out what other climbers said about its physical and mental hurdles. Going during the best climbing season is just as important. For example, June to September is the best season in Europe, while June to August is ideal for Colorado.

2. *PEAK CONDITION*

Being physically fit for the journey is of utmost importance. Jogging, and especially hiking, will give you an important endurance boost that will allow you to stay energetic for longer. Consider lifting weights to give yourself extra arm and leg strength and yoga for flexibility.

Obviously, practicing climbing on an indoor rock wall will teach you several very important skills. The most important result of rock climbing is that it will get you used to heights, hopefully lowering any potential anxiety. A few other important rock climbing skills include: learning to push up with your legs rather than pulling yourself up with your arms, going slow and planning out every move, and knowing when to rest.

3. *WATCH YOUR WEIGHT*

Everything you pack will have to be carried up the mountain by you, so don't plan on taking your Keurig. Take dried, easily stored meals that will last for a long time such as trail mix or jerky. Bring water purification tabs so you don't have to boil water every time you want to drink. In terms of clothing, only pack underwear and socks. Wear lots of light layers, as the clothes on your back should be the only ones brought with you, and you must be prepared for all kinds of weather. Obviously a winter coat is necessary in cooler climates, but a light rain jacket is a must even in sunny weather. The micro-climates of mountains can change without warning, and you don't want to be unprepared and hundreds of miles from civilization when a storm hits. For first aid, pack a small kit that includes bandages and iodine tabs for easy disinfection.

4. *SLEEP LOW, NOT HIGH*

In general, humans don't do well at high altitudes and suffer from an array of potentially lethal problems that go beyond a fear of heights. If you're climbing a mountain fewer than 10,000 feet this shouldn't be an issue, but it's always important to remember high altitudes can cause dizziness (which can cause you to make a deadly mistake) and even pulmonary edema (difficulty breathing because of fluid in the lungs). As a rule of thumb, set up a camp at a lower altitude. You can always climb high but get down to a lower altitude when it's time to rest for the night.

HOW TO MAKE ROPE OUT OF NATURAL MATERIALS

 OU CAN'T underestimate the quality of good rope. And while a cord of survival rope should always be with you when traveling through the great outdoors, accidents happen and sometimes you may need to fashion your own out of nothing but what Mother Nature has provided. Here's how to keep from unraveling under pressure.

1. *GATHER SOME GRASS*

For the purposes of making rope, plants consist of two materials—starch and fiber. Fiber is your friend, the tough material you can twist into workable material. Starch is the enemy. Its presence in any finished rope is sure to weaken it (and possibly cause it to snap at an inopportune moment).

With that in mind, search for dead plants (dead = less starch) that have a lot of fiber in their stalks such as milkweed or dogsbane. While those plants will give you the strongest fiber, any type of long grass can do in a pinch, assuming you aren't crafting a safety harness for scaling Mt. Everest or something similarly critical.

2. *POUND IT OUT*

Now that you have plants chock-full of fiber, you need to separate that fiber from the rest of the plant. Place the plants/stems on a flat surface and use a smooth rock (or any other heavy object) to gently crush the material lengthwise, which splits everything open without risking

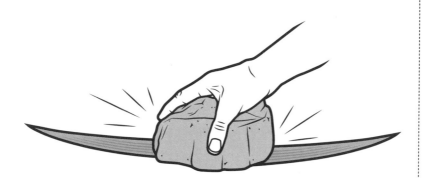

cutting the fibers. Now use a knife, your hands, a sharp rock, etc. to gently separate the string fibers from the outer shell of whatever you just broke apart.

3. *MAKE IT FLEXIBLE*

While you may be fortunate enough to happen upon fiber that's pliable enough to work with straight away, you likely will need to soften the material first. Take the stringy, tough strands of fiber you've now collected and rub them either between your hands or against your thigh for friction to work its magic. The fiber strands should be thin and fluffy before you start fashioning them into a rope.

4. *DO THE TWIST*

Take two bundles of fiber and tie them together on the top with a simple knot. Alternatively, you can take a single bundle and twist it until it kinks up and forms a loop. Make sure the sides are unequal in length, as this will make for a stronger rope if you have to splice additional material into one side

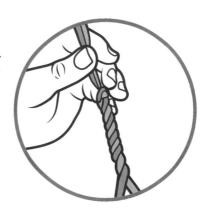

and then the next (splices should be staggered between the two bundles for optimal rope strength). Now hold the top of the bundle (by the knot or loop) with your nondominant hand. There should now be two lengths of fiber bundles, one longer than the other. Lay the strands across your lap or onto a flat surface. Grab the strand farthest from you and twist or roll it away from you between the thumb and fingers of your dominant hand until the fiber tightens. Once it does, hold it tightly between your thumb and forefinger. Use the remaining fingers of your dominant hand to pull the bundle closest to you under and in front of the tightened one, essentially causing them to swap positions. Let go of the original bundle, grab the one that's now farthest from you and tighten it in the same way you did the first one. Bring the original bundle forward just as before, swapping their positions once again. Repeat this process again and again.

5. *TIE ONE OFF*

When you have wrapped almost the entire length of the fiber you're working with, you have a choice. Either tie the strands off at the end to make your finished product, or take a new length of fiber of similar thickness to the one you're working with and splice it into your original length of fiber to form a longer rope by laying new strands of fiber over the ones you were using and continue twisting and wrapping as you were. That's all there is to it, partner.

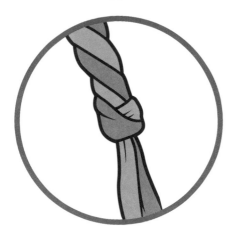

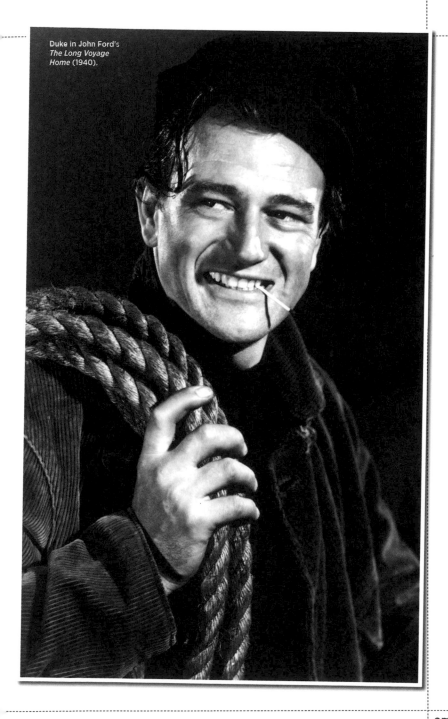

Duke in John Ford's
*The Long Voyage
Home* (1940).

HOW TO MAKE A BOW AND ARROW

 HEN YOU FIND YOURSELF in a survival situation, you need to do everything you can to stay safe and keep your belly full. A bow and arrow, one of humanity's earliest and most reliable weapons, can be a lifesaver when all seems lost. It may not be the simplest of tools to fashion out of the wilderness, but once you've crafted your bow and arrow, you've taken a large leap toward asserting your dominance over the deadly wilderness.

1. *ENSURE THE WOOD IS GOOD*

You can't just grab any old branch off the ground and expect to transform it into a working weapon of the wilderness. The wood for your bow needs to be both flexible and durable, while also free of deformities such as knots. One way to test the wood is to take a small twig and bend it. Did it spring back into shape quickly? Then you have a winner. Find a sapling or large branch of quality wood about 6 feet in length—this will be your bow.

2. *FINDING THE CURVE*

Take your piece of wood, place one end on the ground and loosely hold

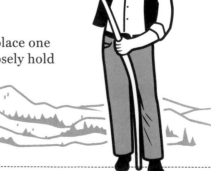

the other end with your hand. Now take your free hand and push forward in the center of the wood until it rotates. It should stop on the natural bend on the piece of wood. The side of the wood facing you is called the belly, while the side facing away from you is called the back. Take dead aim at the center of the wood, and then using a knife or sharp rock, cut a mark around three inches above and below the center—the area in between these marks is your handhold.

3. *WHITTLE AWAY*
Bend your piece of wood/ bow stave again, and make note of which areas refuse to budge. Whittle away those areas on the sides and belly only until the whole piece is flexible—never the back, as that will compromise the strength of the bow. Keep whittling until the upper and lower parts of the bow have roughly the same curvature.

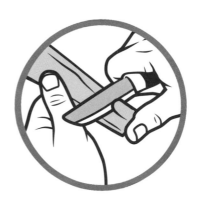

4. *NOTCH AND STRING IT*
Toward the tip of each end of the bow, cut at a 45 degree angle beginning on the sides and running toward the belly side of the bow, pointed at the handhold. Next, take whatever material you are using for bowstring (whether synthetic material such as shoelaces

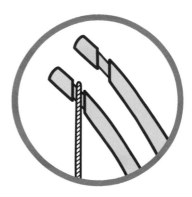

or twine/rope you made in the wild) and tie it securely to each knot, stringing the bow. Make sure your bow string is slightly shorter than the bow is long, as you want the string to be taut. Test your bow by pulling back on the string—both ends should bend evenly. If not, that means you need to whittle more wood away from the inflexible end.

5. *STRAIGHT AND ARROW*

Now that you have a bow, you need something to shoot. Look for straight shoots from nearby trees about .25 to .5 inches thick. The length of the arrow's shaft should be roughly three inches more than the distance you are able to pull back your bowstring (called its draw). Most importantly, arrows need to be absolutely straight. One surefire method of getting straight arrows is by building a fire and holding the individual shoots over the flame until they are heated but not scorched. Then pull up on the shoot until it is straightened, helping ensure your arrows will fly true. If there are any feathers lying about or, more likely, pine needles, gather them together and tie some in a bundle around the end of the arrow opposite of the point—it will help keep your projectile flying straight.

6. *STAY SHARP*

While it would be nice to have arrowheads, you're in a survival situation—simply sharpening one end of your arrow into a point will suffice.

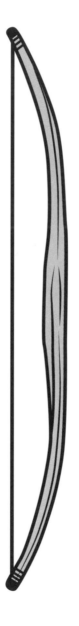

On the other end, cut a small notch that the bowstring will snugly fit into. Now you've got everything you need to bag some big game (or at least something to keep you from starving to death).

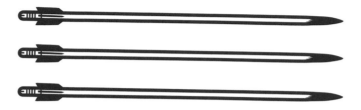

HOW TO HUNT GAME

OK. You have yourself a dandy new bow and arrow—now it's time to put them to good use in getting you some dinner! At its most basic, hunting is simply remaining undetected by prey until it's too late for your dinner to escape. You won't have access to camo gear or scent maskers that you might bring with you on a weekend hunting trip, but you can still follow the time-honored basics of woodcraft to help give you an edge over a rabbit or doe. First of all, pick the proper time to hunt, which for most animals will be either in the early hours of the morning or during dusk, when many creatures roam in search of water and food themselves. Try and spot any tracks in the dirt or mud nearby—animals typically travel along the path of least resistance, so a trail used once will likely see repeat traffic, both by the original animal and others. Once you spot your prey, move carefully into a position where you can take your shot, and then let loose with the arrow! With skill and some luck, you'll be chowing down on meat soon.

HOW TO CATCH A FISH WITH YOUR HANDS

 ISHING IS a tradition any lover of the outdoors should partake in at least once. The battle between man and fish is a noble one, celebrating and strengthening our ingenuity and resolve against a determined opponent. But even more impressive than reeling in the big one? Snatching it with your bare hands out of what it thinks to be a safe space. Just a word of warning—you may feel an urge to bite straight into the animal as you get carried away by the sheer badassery of your deed, but try and show some restraint.

1. *KNOW YOUR ENEMY*
When selecting your quarry, make sure you're aware that some fish fight back harder than others. Catfish, for example, are known to inflict serious cuts to people who pluck them from their waters. Sharks are...sharks. It's difficult enough to haul in a fish barehanded without having to worry about losing an arm in the process.

2. *GET IN POSITION*
Even though the fish are in the water, that doesn't mean your whole body needs to be. Instead, find a bank hanging over a deep, slow-moving tide. Lean down and dip your arm into the water until it's just above your elbow. Then, be still and wait. Fish don't go near objects that are warmer than the water and its surroundings, so you have to wait for your arm to stop radiating heat. After about 15 minutes, fish will have

trouble telling the difference between your arm and underwater vegetation.

3. *LURE LIKE A WORM*

Use your index finger to lure your fish. Mimic worm movements by wiggling it. This makes your finger look like an insect or other small creature and will lure the fish into your clutches.

4. *GRAB 'EM BY THE GILLS*

Once the fish is in your range, snatch it! You have to be quick and aim your fingers under its gills, where you'll find a good amount of bone and cartilage. Holding onto the fish there will make it easier to keep him from slipping away as he begins to thrash.

HOW TO CATCH FISH WITH A SPEAR

If you would rather land your fish with a spear, grab hold of a spear (if possible) or just sharpen a long stick on one end if you are in a pinch. With your spear in hand, step into the shallows of the water. Wait for any fish you may have disturbed with your movements to settle down and resume their normal fish business of swimming and ignoring you (it should go without saying it's important to remain still if you want the fish to calm down). Now all that's left to do is to skewer that fish with your spear.

Simple, right? Wrong. If you remember third grade science, you should know about the law of refraction, which means because of how light bends when it enters water, the fish you are seeing through the surface is actually in a different position than what your eyes are telling you (think of how a drinking straw looks through a glass of clear water). Your rule of thumb should be to aim below the fish you see in order to make deadly contact. Now congratulate yourself on a successful hunt!

HOW TO CAST A FISHING LINE

HE MODERN SPINNING REEL, introduced in 1948, is a versatile rod that can be used in all kinds of situations—if you know how to cast it. This technique is simple but may require practice to get it just right.

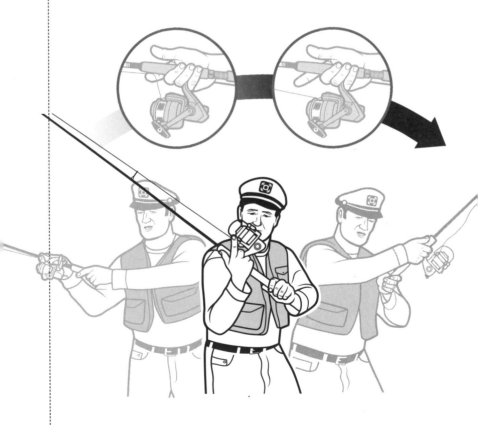

1. *USE A FIRM GRIP*
Using your dominant hand, grasp the rod
around the reel seat. If you just baited the hook,
make sure your hands are clean and dry—you don't
want the rod slipping out of your hands.

2. *ADJUST THE LINE*
You want your bait to be at the ideal distance for
casting, which is 6–12 inches from the rod tip. Either
reel in or feed out the line as needed.

3. *SECURE THE LINE*
Placing your other hand just past the reel, use your
index finger to press the line to the rod. That line
shouldn't be going anywhere just yet!

4. *RELEASE THE LINE*
Open the reel bail, and get ready to cast.

5. *SWING IT BACK*
With your index finger still on the line, swing the rod
back past your shoulder...

6. *CAST THE LINE*
...then sweep the rod forward, releasing your index
finger as you extend your arm. If things don't go as
planned, simply reel it back in and try again. After
a few tries, you'll figure out exactly when to release
your finger and be able to cast a line that would
make Duke proud.

HOW TO COOK WITH AN OPEN FLAME

HETHER IT'S A family camping trip or a survival situation that calls for building a fire and feeding your crew, it's important to get acquainted with three methods of using an open flame (i.e. no grill rack is available) so you don't char your chow. The good news is most of the preparation takes no time at all—just place a few items in your emergency go-bag (p. 70) if you feel you'll be away for long enough to have to cook: Most of the work is done, just like that. Ideally, the hardest part about cooking over an open flame should be building the right fire (which you can learn all about on p. 8). With these three simple methods, any wilderness cookery problem can be overcome.

1. *COME WITH A CORRECT CONTAINER*
A small metal container with a cover is an ideal addition to your camping supplies and emergency kit because it can be packed with other useful items and won't take up too much space. A pot is ideal for survival cooking, as stewing game keeps all the fats and nutrients from dripping off into the fire. When your next meal is uncertain, getting everything you can from a catch is essential, and a makeshift stew is your best option. Simply rake some hot coals out of the fire but near enough to get residual heat and place the pot directly into the coals until the meat is done.

2. *YOUR HUNGER GETS FOILED AGAIN*
Wrapping food in tin foil is similar in theory to the container method and a great way to cook things like

vegetables with an open flame. Both use hot coals rather than direct flame-to-food contact and both serve to protect the food from ash and dirt while preserving its nutritional content. Especially useful for things like baked potatoes, a simple roll of tin foil could be one of the most useful camping items you remember to pack. Simply wrap your food in foil and place directly on the hot coals.

3. *WHEN IN DOUBT, DO A SPIT TAKE*

If you're really in a pickle and you've got neither a fireproof container nor some foil, you can cook your dinner like a true pioneer by cutting two boughs to approximately equal length. Cut off all the twigs and branches except for a Y-shaped joint—created by a smaller branch as it juts from the main bough—on each. Dig the poles into the ground beside your fire pit, far enough away that they won't risk being burnt.

Next, find a stick long enough to cross the fire pit and rest in the branches over the flame. Tie your dinner to the stick and place it across the two branches. Rotate periodically over the flame to ensure even cooking.

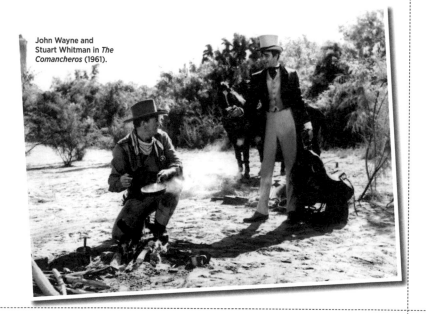

John Wayne and Stuart Whitman in *The Comancheros* (1961).

HOW TO REPEL MOSQUITOES

HE ANIMAL responsible for the most misery in humanity's history isn't the lion, tiger or even the bear—it's the humble mosquito. These little bloodsuckers spread an arsenal of diseases causing debilitation and death, so don't think wanting to avoid a mosquito bite is a sign of weakness. It's an indication of your intelligence as an independent man of action ready to combat any threat. Here's how to keep these potentially deadly pests away from you.

1. *FIGHT WITH FASHION*
Although this isn't a natural repellent, it's a very important tip that can help you in any case, even if you brought your repellent. Make sure you dress appropriately. Cover your arms and legs in order to protect yourself from mosquitoes. Mosquitoes are attracted to darker colors, so try to wear lighter colors while camping. They're also not able to see yellow, which makes it a useful fashion choice.

2. *FIRE IS YOUR FRIEND*
Most people believe the smoke from a campfire contains magical properties that drive mosquitoes away. Most people are wrong. Your run-of-the-mill smoke from normal kindling won't do much to deter the insect, but if you happen upon some eucalyptus or citriodora plants, throw them into the inferno—the smoke from these plants helps keep the bugs away, according to certain studies.

3. *SMELL LIKE A MAN*

Do you emerge from a shower smelling like a Valentine's Day bouquet? Mosquitoes are attracted to strong sweet scents, so avoid washing up with fragrant soaps and shampoos. Just don't avoid bathing altogether, or else it won't just be insects that avoid you.

HOW TO TREAT A MOSQUITO BITE

This should be simple, right? Just scratch away! That's an excellent method if you want to develop a nasty infection, but most of us would rather avoid a trip to the hospital because we couldn't keep our dirty nails from scratching open our skin.

First, if you want to effectively combat the itchiness of a mosquito bite, it's helpful to know exactly what causes them to itch to begin with. When a little bloodsucker sticks her (and it is always a her) needle-like proboscis into your unprotected skin, she starts injecting her saliva into you, which helps expand your blood vessels and prevents the blood from clotting. A couple of hours after she has had her fill and flown away (hopefully finding her end at the palm of your hand), your body's immune system kicks in and causes an inflammatory response to the mosquito's spit. This reaction is what causes those signature, itchy red welts.

It stands to reason that the only remedies worth a damn are those that fight the inflammatory response. Which also means coating yourself in lavender oil or rubbing salt or any other method from an old wives' tale isn't going to stop that itch. So what does? Steroids. Not the kind your high school football coach warned you to steer clear of, but rather the kind that comes in a topical, over-the-counter cream. Rubbing this cream on the bite should lessen the itching as the steroids constrict the blood vessels and lessen the inflammation. If your bite swells up to the size of a small child's head or people greet you by asking "Dear God, what is that thing on your arm?" you should probably make your way to the doc's.

HOW TO BUILD A SNOW SHELTER

 N IGLOO might be the ideal snow-bound shelter to craft, but unfortunately not everyone has the time, energy or necessary companionship to complete such an ambitious task in a survival situation. For emergency know-how, there is no shelter better in the snow than the humble quinzee. Essentially a hollowed out mound of snow, there's a bit more to it than just digging a hole.

1. *GET TO SHOVELIN'*
Create a mound of snow 7'-8' tall and big enough around to fit about two people. Mix snow of different temperatures—some fresh and wet, some that has been left on the frozen ground for a while—to facilitate the hardening process, called "sintering" when you're referencing snow. Form your mound into a dome and let it sinter for at least 90 minutes.

2. *MAKE SOME MEASURING STICKS*
Cut approximately two dozen sticks into 2-foot-long pieces. Stick them at regular intervals through the outer part of your mound, making sure they're completely embedded. During the next step, these will serve to let you know when to stop digging so your walls won't be too thin.

3. *DIG!*
On the downhill side of your domed mound, dig an entrance tunnel about 3 feet high, and begin

CAN I DRINK SNOW TO SURVIVE?

As you know, snow is simply frozen water. Which means in a survival situation, that barren frozen wasteland is really a sea of drinkable water, right? Yes and no. If you have a fistful of snow, a lot of it is actually air, which means you would have to shove an obscene amount of the stuff into your mouth in order to get enough hydration to make a difference in a survival situation. Besides being an inefficient way of taking in water, eating snow also has a cooling effect on your core temperature. To avoid being a well-hydrated person suffering from hypothermia, figure out a way to melt the snow into water first before gulping it down. Obviously if you are able to build a fire and boil the snow in a vessel of some sort, that's the best way of going about it. If you can't get a fire going, you can gather snow into some sort of container and leave that out in the sun during the day, where the heat will hopefully melt the frozen water and give you something to quench your thirst.

hollowing out your mound from the top down. When you reach the measuring sticks, smooth out the wall and ceiling with the side of your shovel or any flat object. These will ensure your walls are two feet thick, more than enough to protect from the elements as well as cave-ins. Leave about a foot of snow on the ground inside the quinzee.

4. *FINISHING TOUCHES*
Dig a small trench down the middle of the quinzee through the remaining foot of snow, all the way to the entrance. This will encourage cold air to leave the shelter regularly as well as create two elevated "bed" areas. Be sure to change into warm, dry clothes after building your quinzee to prevent hypothermia, because you'll have worked up a sweat.

HOW TO RECOGNIZE VENOMOUS SNAKES

EFORE VENTURING out into the great outdoors, every man should check and see what venomous snakes might be lurking. The Centers for Disease Control and Prevention estimates between 7,000 and 8,000 people get bitten by venomous snakes in the U.S. per year. This guide is going to help make sure you're not one of them.

When you're trudging through the undergrowth in the forest, you should already be looking at the ground to ensure you aren't walking through poison oak or ivy. Just add snakes to your list as something to watch out for. Most venomous snakes do not go out of their way to attack humans. If you accidentally step on one though, they're not going to be happy about it. Snakes are the kings of camouflage, and they purposefully stay still when they hear movement, which is why you need to be extra vigilant. But for those times where you aren't sure if you're looking at a harmless critter or one that could put you down for good, these tips should help sort you out. That said—better safe than dead. If you're in doubt, steer clear.

1. *DO SOME RESEARCH*
There are about 20 species of venomous snakes in America. It's unlikely you're going to encounter all of them unless you're pulling a Gump and crisscrossing

the country by foot. If you're walking around the Northeast, you're not going to run across the vibrant Western coral snake, but you should be looking out for the Copperhead. It ranges as far north as New York State and as far west as Nebraska.

2. OBSERVE THE SNAKE'S MARKINGS AND SHAPE (IF YOU HAVE TIME)

Venomous snakes often have triangle-shaped heads, which they flatten when feeling threatened. They also often have heat-sensing pits on the sides of their nostrils, but you probably don't want to get that close to a threatening reptile. If you can't get a good look at the snake's head, you should look for a rattle on the snake's tail, as every type of rattlesnake is venomous. But just because you don't see (or hear) a tell-tale rattle, don't let down your guard—some rattlesnakes lose their rattlers through age or injury. Other snakes, notably the coral snake, come with a popular rhyme to help you differentiate it from its harmless look-alike, the Scarlet Kingsnake: "Red to yellow, kill a fellow; red to black, venom lack."

3. SWIMMING STYLE

There are a few types of venomous snakes that swim, including the Yellow-Bellied Sea Snake and the Water Moccasin, aka Cottonmouth. Instead of spending your time worrying about what lurks deep in the water, keep your eyes on the surface. If you see a snake swimming on the top of the water, just get out of its way.

4. ASSUME THE WORST

While the above information is sound, there's also an easy way to deal with identifying venomous snakes— just assume every snake you see slithering packs a potentially lethal bite. That way if you're surprised, you won't pay for it with your life.

HOW TO RECOGNIZE POISONOUS PLANTS

OTHER NATURE paints a colorful landscape in the wilderness with flowers, grasses and plants of almost every shape and hue, adding to the pleasure of spending time in the great outdoors. However, many of these plants are best observed from a distance; woe to the hiker or camper who beds down in a patch of poison ivy or treats the berries of a nearby tree like free samples from your local supermarket. Your best protection against accidental poisoning is knowing the plants specific to the area, usually gleaned from a local guidebook, but here are a couple of general guidelines that should keep you safe.

1. *BASIC MATH*

The old adage "Leaves of three, let it be!" isn't the most scientific but can help you avoid poison ivy and poison oak—though some species of both contain more than three leaves. And other plants such as poison sumac can have as many as 13 leaves but still give you an itchy rash upon contact. That said, avoiding any plant with three leaves is a good rule to follow—just don't let it be the only one.

2. *BROAD BAN*

If you're trying to determine if a plant is a suitable candidate to include in a survival situation salad, it's better to play it safe than sorry. After all, you can go quite a long time without any food, but a bout of poisoning can leave you incapacitated or worse. Keep away from any plants that produce a milky, white sap when broken, as well as any that look hairy, have white berries or shiny leaves. And, steer clear of mushrooms and berries you can't confidently identify.

3. *GET GRASS*
While maybe not the most appealing meal, all grasses are safe to eat. You shouldn't just swallow them whole, but chew the leaves and swallow the (albeit meager) juice they produce. Bon appetit!

HOW TO TEST IF A PLANT IS EDIBLE (KIND OF)

As mentioned in the advice on this page, you are far better off avoiding the ingestion of any plants you don't absolutely know are non-toxic. If for whatever reason you have no choice but to chow down on the mysterious-looking flowers nearby, follow these steps to help reduce your chance of eating your last meal.

1. Take all the parts of the plant—the root, the flowers, the leaves, etc.—and separate them from each other. You'll need to test each one individually as some parts of a plant can be toxic while the others are safe.

2. Take a big sniff of what you are testing. Bad odor? That's a pass. Smells strongly of almonds? Yeah, you are holding poison in your hands right now. Don't put that in your mouth, please.

3. Rub the plant on the inside of your arm or your elbow and then wait about a half hour or so. If there is any itching, tingling or irritation then you don't want that plant going down your gullet.

4. Any plant that passes these steps should be boiled if possible. Then take the plant and rub it against your lips to test for irritation or burning. If you don't feel any after 15 minutes, put it in your mouth and hold it in there for a few minutes. Anything that tastes extremely bitter or like dish soap is a no-no.

HOW TO RAISE YOUR BODY TEMPERATURE

HE COLD KILLS. You may think complaining about the cold (even to yourself) is a sign of weakness, but frostbite and hypothermia (defined as your core body temperature falling below 95 degrees) have both claimed more than their fair share of fingers, toes, eyes, ears and lives. When enjoying the great outdoors, you need to do the responsible thing and protect yourself from frigid temperatures. Read on and get smart about warming up.

1. *LAYER UP*

Let's start with two basic facts about heat and cold. Heat is a form of energy generated by the movement of molecules, while cold is merely the absence of that energy. Now that you've passed Physics 101, you should understand the most effective ways of raising your body temperature involve capturing and preserving the heat generated by any nearby source. And you can't very well capture the heat of a fire if you're wearing shorts and a cotton Tommy Bahama shirt in the middle of a tundra. Before venturing out into the cold, put on a pair of long underwear, thick socks and layer up from there. You'll want to pick clothing that traps the heat of your body, which materials such as wool do incredibly well.

2. *HUNKER DOWN*

Another action to take when worried about hypothermia is to seek shelter. Obviously, if you're a short stroll away from a cabin complete with a roaring fire, warm blankets and a space heater, make your way there instead of standing outside in the cold. But even when there's no warm shelter in sight, you should still do everything you can to protect yourself from wind and wetness, the two things that will cause your core body temperature to sink like a stone. Even if it's as primitive as digging a small hole to lie in to avoid the wind, a few degrees can make a vital difference.

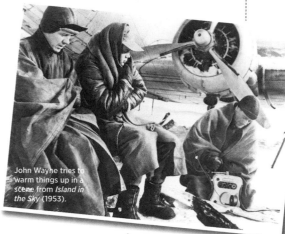

John Wayne tries to warm things up in a scene from *Island in the Sky* (1953).

3. *FRIENDLY FIRE*

A fire will provide you much-needed heat, but you have to balance the advantages of the flame against the energy you'll expend making it. Your body is using calories in an attempt to keep you warm (which you notice as shivering in the beginning stages of hypothermia), and an exhausted person is more likely to get picked off by the cold in a permanent way. If you see a lot of usable fuel in the form of kindling or are carrying with you tools that aid in making a fire, you should make that a priority. Otherwise, you'll have to assess for yourself how much danger you're in and whether the labor of building a fire is the smart move.

If you do build a fire, wrap yourself in as many layers as possible and stay near the flames. Don't ever warm a water bottle or some other vessel in the fire and place it directly on your skin—you don't want a nasty burn. In most cases, your core temperature will raise at a rate of about 3.6 degrees every hour, putting you out of danger.

HOW TO SHARPEN A KNIFE

 IKE A rugged individualist without this book, a knife without a sharp edge is a sad sight to behold. The old adage that a dull knife is more dangerous than a sharp one is borne out of the reality that a dull blade requires you to work twice as hard to cut half as well, and that extra force often leads to injury when the knife skips a tricky knot on a stick or refuses to glide through a chicken leg. Here's how to hone your blade back to shape, even if you don't have all the proper equipment on hand.

1. *TEST IT OUT*

Your first order of business is determining whether your knife actually needs sharpening. Take your blade and carefully run it flat along the outside of your arm toward your hand. If it cuts off arm hair, it should be sharp enough for any other (more useful) task you have in mind for it. If it cuts off your arm, you had the angle wrong—but at least you know it's sharp!

2. *LIKE A ROCK*

If you have a whetstone, a stone made specifically for sharpening knives, get to using it. Grab the knife by the handle with one hand, and gently grab the top of the blade with the other (being mindful not to cut yourself on the edge). Place the knife edge-first at about a 20 degree angle at the top of the stone. Slide the blade down the whetstone, keeping contact between the edge and stone, until you reach the bottom of the stone. Then flip the knife and slide it back up the stone in the same

WHAT TYPE OF KNIFE SHOULD YOU HAVE WITH YOU?

Any knife is better than no knife. However, if you can pick what knife to carry with you in a survival situation, there are some finer points to consider.

1. Fixed blade knives are always going to be stronger than their foldable counterparts. Sure, you do sacrifice portability and packing space, but the trade-off is a blade that is far less likely to snap back on you when cutting through a thick branch.

2. The size of the knife should be at least 4" in length, and preferably longer if you think you are going to need to use it for some heavy-duty construction. The longer the blade, the easier it is to work with larger pieces of wood.

3. Carbon steel knives may be prone to rust, but they are sharper and easier to keep sharp than their stainless steel brethren. But they're also pricier.

manner. Continue doing this until the knife is sharp enough for your liking.

What if you forgot to pack your whetstone? Look around for a rock with a smooth, flat surface that also has a little bit of grit to it similar to a whetstone and use it the same way you would use the real McCoy.

3. *LOVE YOUR LEATHER*

While not anywhere near as effective as sharpening with a rock, you can strop the blade with a leather belt if needed. Take off your belt and hook the buckle to something solid so you can keep it taut when you tug on it. With your other hand, hold the knife to the belt's surface at a similar angle you would use for a whetstone. Again, make the same motions you would with a whetstone, and you'll at least have gotten rid of deformities on the blade's edge, helping it cut a little cleaner.

HOW TO MAKE A TRAVOIS

HEN YOU'RE out in the great outdoors, you may encounter a situation where you need to move something heavier than your own brute strength can manage. But don't fret—after all, you've been blessed with brains as well as brawn, so take advantage of the traditions of old and outthink the problem. The travois is a simple sled used by the American Indians of the Great Plains to transport all manner of things too heavy to heap on the shoulders, and it's just as reliable today as in days past.

1. *FIND YOUR WOOD*
   Search for a sapling or fallen branch of sturdy wood you can cut down to size for your travois. The longer a travois's poles are, the easier it is to carry your load. However, a 20-foot-long pole would be both extremely heavy to drag as well as unwieldy. Aim for two pieces of wood between 8 and 10 feet in length. Also, gather three to four other shorter pieces of wood that will serve as the support between the two poles. Again, don't overdo it here: more wood = more weight.

2. *LASH OUT*
   Take the two poles and use either your belt, shoelace or suitable natural material at hand (see page 34) to lash two ends of the poles together. Then take the shorter pieces of wood and lash them across the base of the two poles in a ladder shape, completing the travois.

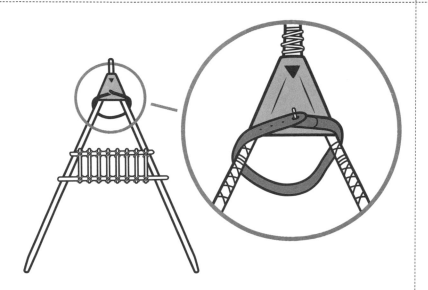

3. *GET TO DRAGGING*

Place your load on the base of the travois, making sure your sled can bear the weight. Then grab the two poles at the top of the travois and place them over your shoulder or at your hips (whichever is more comfortable) to drag it with maximum efficiency.

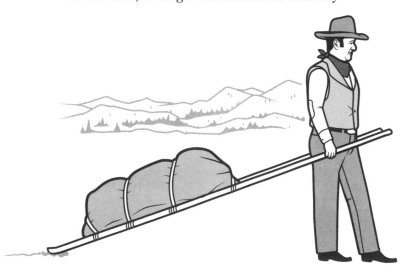

HOW TO
TREAD WATER

N 1953'S *HONDO,* John Wayne's titular character helps a young boy learn to swim the best way he knows how—by chucking him into a nearby river. While we hesitate to argue with Duke's teaching methods, it's probably best to know some of the fundamentals of how to stay afloat in water before diving (or being thrown) in headfirst. But should you find yourself in water either of your own or someone else's volition, it helps to know what to do with yourself in order to get back to shore. Treading water is a vital skill, particularly if shore is an unswimmable distance away.

1. *FEEL THE RHYTHM*
There are plenty of different ways to tread water, but what they all have in common is an emphasis on steady motions that don't waste energy. Keep your cool and avoid making jerky, thrashing motions that will only tire you out and send you sinking.

2. *SWEEP AND FLUTTER*
One easy way to successfully tread water involves what is called "sculling" with your arms while your feet flutter back and forth to keep you afloat. With your arms completely submerged in water, sweep them in a large semi-circle in front of you with the palms facing outward, as if you were trying to part the water in front toward either side of you. Then bring your arms and hands together as if you were going to clap them, stopping just shy of contact. You should keep repeating this movement for the duration of your time in the water.

At the same time, you should keep your legs straight with your toes pointed down. Move each leg back and forth in a smooth motion, paying attention to the position of your feet to make sure they stay pointed down. Together, these motions should keep your head above water where you want it.

3. *GET BACK*

If you need a brief breather, float on your back with your legs and arms still submerged in the water. Bend your arms at the elbow and keep your hands flat, palms facing down. Paddle those hands up and down in a smooth motion while your feet gently kick back and forth. Arch your back slightly and breathe slowly, holding your breath as long as is comfortable. This gives your core a break from staying upright at the cost of spending a little more energy moving your arms and legs.

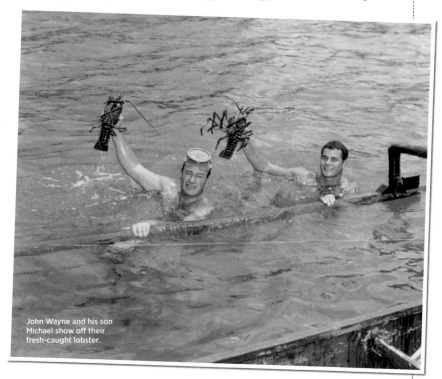

John Wayne and his son Michael show off their fresh-caught lobster.

HOW TO CLEAN, SCALE AND GUT A FISH

HETHER YOU CAUGHT the fish yourself or bought it whole from the supermarket, plan to clean it within an hour or two, keeping it cold and wet until you're ready to do so. This is also an activity best suited for the outdoors—gutting a fish is a messy process but well worth the work.

1. *GATHER YOUR SUPPLIES*
On a newspaper-covered table, set out a bucket for the fish parts, a sharp cutting knife, a container for the cleaned fish and gloves (optional).

2. *SCALE THE FISH*
Holding the fish firmly by the tail, use your knife to scrape the scales off, working from the tail toward the gills. Be careful not to exert too much pressure— you don't want to gash the fish.

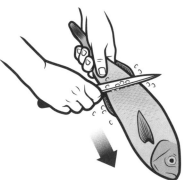

3. *RINSE THE FISH*
Once you've cleared the scales from both sides, rinse the fish with clean water. If using a hose or spigot, be careful not to use too much pressure, as fish meat is delicate.

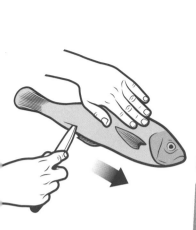

4. *MAKE THE MAIN CUT*

Insert a fillet knife at the base of the fish near the tail, and draw the knife toward the head, splitting the fish. If you're working with a small fish, you can hold it down on its side with one hand while cutting it; a larger fish should be placed on its back.

5. *SPREAD THE CAVITY OPEN*

Using your fingers, open up the cut you've just made. Reach in with your other hand and pull out the entrails, placing them in your parts bucket.

6. *RINSE THE CAVITY*

Rinse the inside of the fish with water, and then the outside once more.

7. *REMOVE THE HEAD*

This step is optional. Some fish are cooked with the heads on, but many pan-sized fish are not. If removing, cut the head off from behind the gills.

HOW TO TIE SPECIALTY KNOTS

 OPE IS at once one of the most useful survival tools you can have and also one of those that takes the most practice to perfect. If you're like most modern folks, tying your shoelaces is as close to knot-tying merit badge territory as you'll get. But bunny ears simply won't cut it in the wild. A good knot can save a life in the wilderness, whether it's protecting you from wind, water, a fall or working as a component keeping your shelter up or your traps full. For clarity, the "working end" of a rope is the portion you're going to be looping around things, while the "standing end" is the portion that leads to the rest of the rope.

SQUARE KNOT

A square knot is used to tie two lengths of rope together for extension or strength-enhancing purposes.

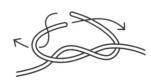

Hold the ends of the ropes you wish to tie together. Pass one end over and then under the other. Repeat the motion and pull tight, the same as you would to tie a pair of boots—just remember to skip the loops.

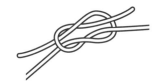

CLOVE HITCH

Also known as a double hitch, the clove hitch is

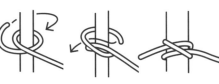

a quick, temporary knot commonly used for securing a line on a post. Easily cast off when not in need, it won't hold permanently but is great for short-term heavy lifting both literal and figurative.

To make this knot, pass the end of the rope around a post. Continue over the standing end and around the pole a second time. Thread the end under itself and pull tight.

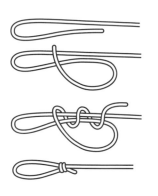

SLIPKNOT

A slipknot, which gets its name because the simple knot can slide easily up and down a length of rope, is useful for creating an adjustable loop. A slipknot will add pressure around the object with a simple tug, and can be just as easily undone.

Make a loop by doubling the rope back on itself. Pass one end of the rope back up, forming a figure eight. Wrap that same end around the double lines of rope a few times and pull tight. Slide the knot up or down to adjust the size of your loop.

TIMBER HITCH

The Timber Hitch is useful for dragging logs and easily comes loose when you stop pulling on it. When building a longer-term shelter, it's an important knot to know as it will save you time and energy better spent keeping yourself alive than untying knots.

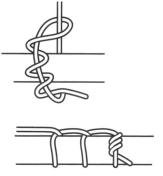

To make this knot, pass the working end of a rope around an object and take a turn around the standing end. Tuck the working end back around itself three times with the lay of the rope.

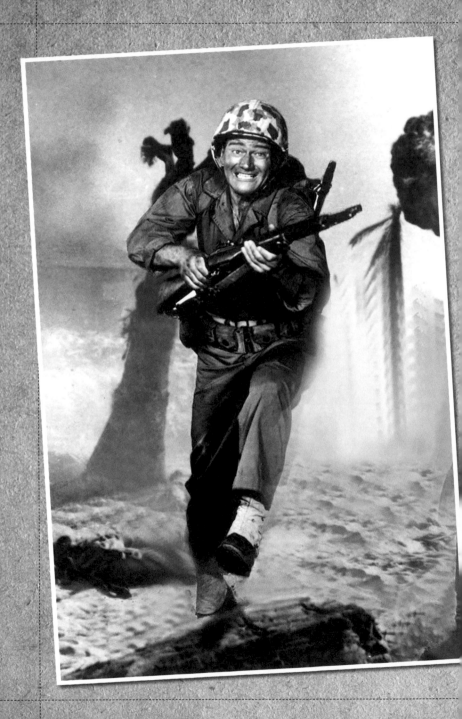

EMERGENCY TACTICS

BE PREPARED FOR ANYTHING AND EVERYTHING LIFE THROWS AT YOU

HOW TO PACK AN EMERGENCY BAG

OR SOME, THE MOTTO "Be Prepared" is more than just good advice: It's a code to live by. Prepping for the worst takes many forms, ranging in mainstream relatability from investing in a life insurance policy to outfitting a fallout shelter with canned goods and radiation-resistant weapons. But anybody can take one step that lies safely in between these two levels of commitment and won't break the bank or require any construction: an emergency preparedness or "bug-out" bag. A good bug-out bag should consist of enough supplies for three full days away from civilization, plus some items that can be useful for longer. This will give you enough to have a leg up on the elements when the stuff hits the fan.

1. *GIMME SHELTER*

Your first priority in a survival situation is finding safe shelter. A lightweight tent marketed toward backpackers, supplemented with a tarp, will go a long way toward protecting you from cold, wind and moisture without adding too much weight to the bag. Disposable chemical hand and foot warmers are also a great (and light) addition.

2. *FIRE IT UP*

Because a well-made fire can make up for inadequacies in other areas—fire can provide warmth if no shelter is available, cook food if you run out of rations and have to hunt, and even purify water if no filtration system is available—fire-making is a vital survival skill. For this reason, you should keep several simple lighters and stormproof matches along with a container of homemade tinder (created by coating cotton balls or dryer lint in petroleum jelly) in your emergency bag.

3. *ESSENTIAL DINING*

A standard amount of water to carry is three liters, which will keep you hydrated and moving for more than the requisite three days. As far as food is concerned, ready-to-eat options like beef jerky, granola or protein bars provide a portable, convenient way to pack energy for your body. Because humans can survive—albeit uncomfortably—without food for much longer than three days, you shouldn't waste too much weight and space by packing a month's worth of food.

4. *PORTABLE PHARMACY*

Beyond packing about a week's worth of any prescription medication you currently need to survive, you should be aware that the biggest medical danger in the wild is blood loss. Base your checklist around items that will help prevent you from bleeding out, such as sterile gauze padding, bandages and a disinfectant such as iodine will go a long way toward making sure you live through a medical mishap.

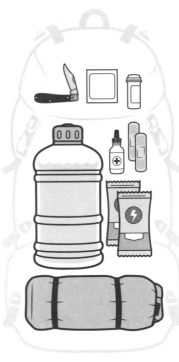

5. *THE BAG ITSELF*

The most essential characteristic your bag should have is that, when full, you can still carry it. So once your bag is relatively laden, take it with you on your morning or evening stroll to get used to the idea of being mobile with the weight.

HOW TO SURVIVE A VENOMOUS SNAKEBITE

HANKS TO YEARS of watching Hollywood heroics (including those found in 1969's *True Grit*), many people think the best cure for a venomous snake bite is to stick a knife in the wound and suck out the gushing mixture of blood and venom. And while one of the crusty old regulars at your local watering hole may swear to that method's efficacy, the truth is he probably mistook a bite from a garden snake for something actually dangerous. And though dying from a snake bite is quite rare these days—only five people out of 7,000-8,000 people bitten by snakes die per year—it's better to be safe than sorry. Here's how to handle a potentially deadly encounter with the real thing.

1. *DON'T GET BITTEN (AGAIN)*
If there's anything worse than suffering a snake bite, it's getting bit by a snake twice. While you'll want to remain as still and calm as possible (an increased heart rate means the venom coursing through your system works even quicker), you need to move out of striking distance from the reptile. If you can, snapping a photo of the snake with your phone (or even just memorizing what it looks like) will help medical workers determine how to best keep you alive, but don't focus on that at the expense of getting to safety.

2. *FOLLOW YOUR HEART*

In order to slow the march of the venom from the bite site to your heart, keep the wound below your heart if possible. If help can come to you, your job is simple—remain calm and wait for your rescuers to whisk you away to safety. But if you have a hike ahead of you, keep the affected area as still as possible when moving. Fashioning an impromptu splint by tying sticks or boards over either side of the wounded area helps, but your number one priority should be getting medical attention.

3. *GET HELP*

There's a line between admirable independence and bone-headed stubbornness we feel comfortable drawing at "walking off a venomous snake bite." The bite of some rattlesnakes, for instance, is loaded with hemotoxins designed to obliterate your blood and soft tissue while also containing neurotoxins which cause side effects such as respiratory paralysis and death. The good news is if administered the proper antivenom by medical professionals, you probably won't lose your life (or a limb). Probably.

HOW TO SURVIVE A BEAR ATTACK

WHEN ENJOYING the splendor of the great outdoors, it behooves you to remember you are very much a visitor in the habitat of some dangerous animals. While bears aren't wandering the woods looking for unwilling participants with whom to re-enact *The Revenant*'s most terrifying scene, these hulking omnivores aren't just a passive part of the scenery posing for your iPhone pic. Should you find yourself on the receiving end of a bear attack, you need to immediately do two things—pray to your god, and remember the tips outlined here.

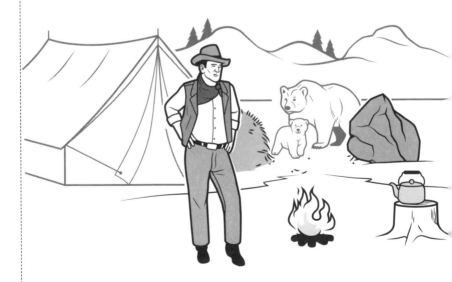

1. *WHAT BEARS WANT*

Your first order of business is trying to determine
why this bear has decided to attack you. The animal's
motive will inform your strategy for making it out alive,
so you need to quickly analyze the situation and act
accordingly to increase your odds of survival. Broadly
speaking, bears of any species (grizzly, black, brown,
Pooh) will attack for one of two reasons—to protect
their cubs or to fill their hairy bellies. Leading up to the
attack, if the bear paws at the dirt, roars and generally
looks scary as hell, that's a strong sign the beast is
actually giving you a warning to back up and clear off.
If the animal makes a beeline toward you with its ears
flat back and isn't wasting time on theatrics...be afraid.
That means the bear means business and doesn't want
to scare you—it wants to eat you.

2. *PASSIVE RESISTANCE*

If you're sure the bear is mounting a defensive attack,
your goal is to convince the beast you aren't a threat.
Curl up in a fetal position on the ground, covering your
head, neck and (most of) your torso to protect it from a
vicious mauling (the miracles of modern medicine can
provide you with a prosthetic leg or arm, but can't yet
give you a new head). If you're flipped onto your back,
roll back onto your stomach, but otherwise you shouldn't
offer any other resistance
to the bear's attack. If all
goes well, the beast will
determine you aren't a
threat to its cubs and
will move on. Make sure
the bear is completely
out of sight before slowly
moving to somewhere
you can get help and/or
medical attention.

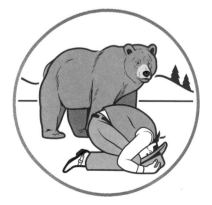

3. *LAST STAND*

On the other hand, there's only one way to deal with a bear that considers you its next meal, and that's fighting back. Playing dead or passive is just going to make the bear's job of eating you easier, so instead make yourself as scary as possible—shout, scream, do whatever you can to convince the bear you aren't just some hairless ape with a relatively high fat-to-muscle ratio. If you're lucky, the bear may decide you are more troublesome than tasty, and break off the attack. But considering you've already encountered a bear that wants to eat you, Lady Luck may not be your best friend right now.

4. *BEAR BATTLE*

So the bear hellbent on eating you wasn't impressed with your intimidating war-cry. On one hand, that's a bummer, but on the other...well let's just say it will be fortunate if you still have two hands at the end of this encounter. While you still do, use them to slap, punch and 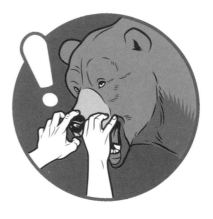 claw the bear in its eyes and nose—its most sensitive areas open to attack. Look, we're not going to sugarcoat it—a grizzly bear can break an adult human's neck with a single swipe of its paw. But if you end up driving the bear away in hand-to-hand combat, you can bask in the knowledge that you accomplished an incredible feat of grit and valor few can match.

HOW TO SURVIVE A SHARK ATTACK

A little-known and also made up fact is that the word "shark" is Latin for "water bear." It would be a shame to survive an encounter with a grizzly one day only to end up in the belly of a great white a week later. Here's what to do if you run (er, swim) into a hungry shark.

1. Stay calm and swim slowly away toward the shore or your boat. Most times, the shark will lose interest as long as you don't make too much of a fuss thrashing about like a panicked, delicious seal.

2. If the shark is still making a beeline for you, switch tactics and make yourself as threatening as possible. Make yourself big by stretching out your arms and legs and make as much noise as you can, and put those screams of terror to good use.

3. The shark may still persist in seeing what you are made of, so don't be afraid to fight it if it gets in range of your punch (well, be afraid). Try and jab the beast in its most sensitive areas, the eyes, the gills and the tip of its nose. Good luck.

HOW TO FIND WATER IN THE DESERT

NOTHING **REAFFIRMS** the fact that our lives revolve around water more than exploring the desert. One of the most impressive feats you can pull off is finding some old-fashioned H_2O in the middle of a barren wasteland, as the cost of failure is usually your life. Take care to follow these tips the next time you're feeling parched on the dunes and realize your waterskins are empty.

1. *PROTECT WHAT YOU HAVE*
The most important thing you can do if you're stuck in the desert is to

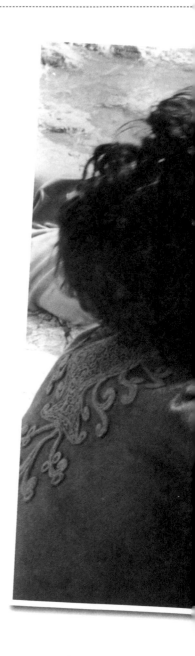

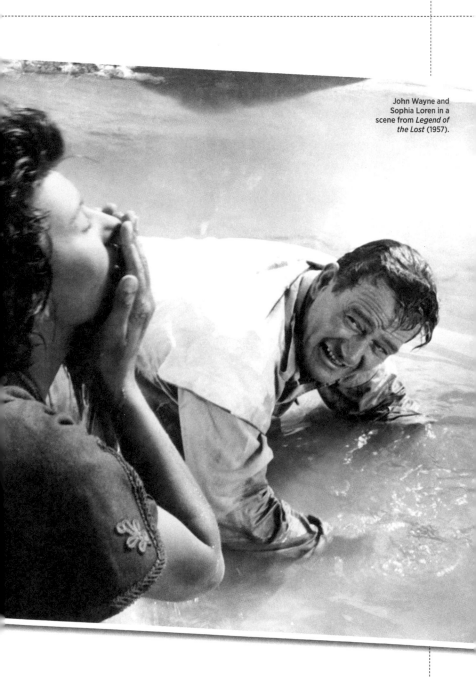

John Wayne and Sophia Loren in a scene from *Legend of the Lost* (1957).

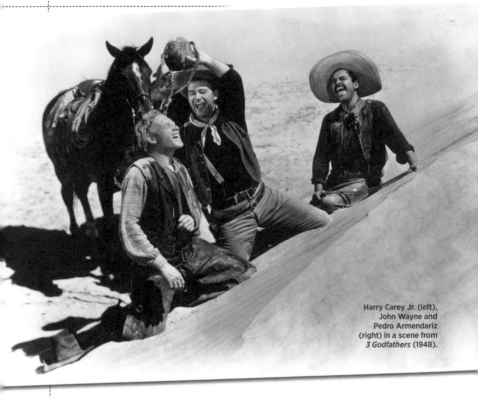

Harry Carey Jr. (left),
John Wayne and
Pedro Armendariz
(right) in a scene from
3 Godfathers (1948).

make sure you conserve water. No matter how urgent
your search for water is, conserving your energy takes
precedence as the onset of dehydration will inhibit your
ability to continue searching. Make sure to find shelter
and shade, especially during the hottest parts of the day.
Keep exertion to a minimum, making sure to keep your
search slow but methodical. Finally, always keep your
skin out of the sun to prevent sweating and sunburn.

2. *FOLLOW THE LOCALS*

Although rare in the desert, a source of fresh water is
your best bet for staying hydrated. A stream or river
is preferable because the constant movement helps
prevent the spread of harmful bacteria. Although it
may seem impossible, there are more than a few tricks

to tracking one down. First, pay attention to animals because they require water as much as you do. Things such as animal tracks in the sand, fly swarms and birds overhead can lead you straight to a freshwater source.

3. *UP AND AT 'EM*

The morning dew can also serve as an emergency water source if you wake up early enough. Try to find cacti before the sun evaporates the dew, using a piece of absorbent fabric (your T-shirt will do in a pinch) to transport the dew once you find it. Half-covered stones may also contain non-evaporated dew if they're turned over early enough in the day.

4. *MAKE LIKE A MOLE*

If you can't find enough available water around you, try searching for it under your feet. Digging for water takes a lot of time and expends a lot of energy, so avoid exerting yourself in direct sunlight by waiting until evening if possible. Dry streams, the ground around the base of mountains or anywhere vegetation is present are good candidates for starting your search. You're looking for a small spot of wet sand, where you can begin digging with a shovel (or more likely, your hands).

Dig until the bottom of your hole is at least a foot below the surface. If the sand is wet you may have found a potential water source (if not, you'll want to move on to avoid wasting precious energy). Get to work making the hole wider until it's about a foot in diameter, then wait a few hours for water to potentially collect. If a pool of water has begun forming, take a piece of cloth and use it to suck up the water and transport it to a container.

HOW TO RATION FOOD AND WATER

T'S EASY TO TAKE FOR GRANTED, but the ability to walk into a store filled with every type of foodstuff imaginable may rank as modern civilization's most remarkable achievement. The glut of sustenance available makes us all the more vulnerable to blunders when forced to ration food and water in an emergency situation. If you find yourself in a tight spot where you need to make do with less, remember the advice below when making the hard decisions.

1. *GET IT WHILE IT'S NOT ROTTEN*

Your first order of business is taking stock of your supply of food and water. Unless you have a working fridge or freezer, perishable food such as uncanned fruits and vegetables, dairy products and meat should be consumed first.

Your water needs depend on a number of factors (someone living in the middle of the Mojave is going to need a lot more fluid than someone in Alaska, for instance), but a useful way to estimate your water need is to take your body weight and divide it in half. The resulting figure is the number of ounces of water you need a day to avoid dehydration. So if you weigh 160 pounds, you will need around 80 ounces of water to be properly hydrated. In a survival situation, you may need to dole out less water, but on average everyone should get at least 40 ounces of water a day—anything less is asking for trouble.

2. *COUNT YOUR CALORIES*

Everyone has daily calorie requirements they need to get

from their food in order to avoid the complications associated with slowly starving to death. These needs are unique to each individual, but in general the minimum needs are:

- *Adult male* 1,700
- *Adult female* 1,328
- *Elderly male* 1,475
- *Elderly female* 1,100
- *Teenage male* 1,655
- *Teenage female* 1,486
- *Youth male* 1,230
- *Youth female* 1,165
- *Baby/toddler* 500–1,000

If your food is prepackaged, as in the case of canned goods, there should be a label telling you how many calories are in each serving size. Otherwise, you'll have to eyeball it using your hand as a guide, remembering the palm of your hand equals about 3 ounces of cooked meat or fish (about 120 calories), while your balled up fist equals about a cup of cooked rice (200 calories) or vegetables (varies depends on the veggie, but a cup of cooked broccoli is about 60 calories).

Ideally you'd want everyone to eat at least their minimum caloric requirement (and more if they are doing any physically taxing work) through a balanced, nutritious diet. But if all you have is a king-sized candy bar to eat...well at least it will be delicious, if not filling.

3. *FOOD ENFORCER*

A somewhat delicate (but very important) rule to establish early is who among you is responsible for dividing up the available food and water into rations. Depending on how close the group is to each other, this could get tricky. Having Mom in charge of the rationing may work great for the family, but if you're stuck with coworkers and task New Guy Mike with the job, he may not have the trust or authority to avoid being ripped apart by his half-starved colleagues. Whoever is placed in charge, he or she needs to have a level head, the respect of the group, and a copy of this book.

HOW TO TREAT A BURN

HETHER YOUR HAND slips when branding your cattle with a red-hot iron (unlikely, but awesome in its way) or you flaunt the laws of thermodynamics by accidentally grasping a pan of cookies fresh from the oven (less awesome, but more likely), there comes a time in every man's life when he needs to treat a burn. Just remember, even the hardiest of rugged individualists knows that when skin is falling off the bone like a delicious rack of ribs, it's time to get emergency medical help. If your burn is hewing closer to shrug-it-off territory, look to the information below for first-aid advice.

1. *TAKE IT OFF .*

The skin you just sizzled is about to swell up like a prized heifer fit for the meat rack, so any jewelry and clothing that could get in the way of treatment should come off so it doesn't become embedded into your flesh.

2. *COOL DOWN (BUT NOT TOO MUCH)*

You're probably not surprised to read one of the first steps in treating a burn is to cool down the damaged area. But you want to be mindful of overdoing it. Don't plunge your burnt hand (or whatever) into a bucket full of ice or in frigid water from the tap. Instead, cool (or even warm) water works best to lower the temperature of the damaged area without harming the surrounding tissue. About 15 to 30 minutes immersed in water should do the trick.

3. *THAT'S A WRAP*

If the burned part of your skin is covered in unbroken blisters you suspect will stay unbroken (i.e. not on the bottom of your foot), leave the burn be. The goo in a blister is the body's way of healing itself. However, if there are open,

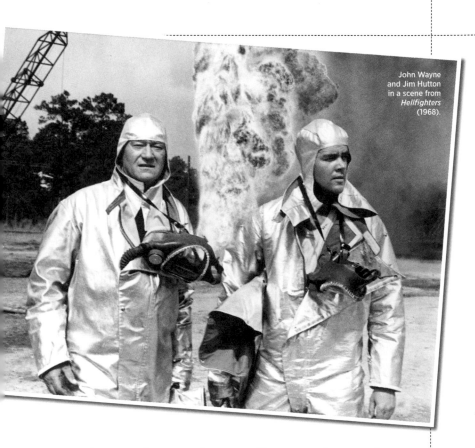

weeping sores from your burn, you'll want to take care of
that. Ideally, you want to loosely wrap the affected area with
a non-adhesive bandage, which you'll change as soon as it
gets wet or soiled. If you want, put a thin layer of petroleum
jelly or aloe vera on the burn to prevent it from drying
out, but don't smear on creams, butter, lotions, etc. You'll
be doing more harm than good by irritating what is now
extremely sensitive skin.

4. *SEEK MEDICAL ATTENTION*
If the burns cover large swaths of your body, have created
large blisters or you suspect there are signs of infection, do
yourself a favor and see a doctor—you don't want to wind up
with sepsis.

HOW TO TREAT FROSTBITE

EMEMBER HOW AS A CHILD your mother fussed over your choice of layering (or lack thereof) every time the temperature dropped below 60? She may have been a bit overzealous, but if you can count to 20 using your fingers and toes, you should thank her for keeping you safe from frostbite. While the name sounds folksy, frostbite occurs when the temperature of any of your extremities drops so low the skin and tissue underneath freezes, causing all sorts of problems. If you find yourself feeling the chill, follow this advice to make sure your future high-fives aren't high-threes.

1. *STOP AND ASSESS*
Take a good, hard look at the damaged area (now is not the time to be squeamish) to see what you're dealing with. Is the skin red and sore? Painful as that is, you should be jumping for joy because you just have frostnip, the easily reversible precursor to frostbite. If you're able to warm the area and protect it from exposure, you'll be fine.

When you find yourself in a situation where you can't shelter your vulnerable bits from the frigid temperatures, you may notice the skin of the affected area looking waxy or taking on a white-greyish hue. This is a sign the frostbite has damaged the deeper layers of tissue beneath the skin's surface. If you suspect your frostbite is anywhere approaching the moderate to severe end of the scale and you're no more than two hours away from a hospital, head there and don't bother with the steps below. Anyone not so fortunate should keep reading to keep themselves from losing a finger or toe (or worse).

2. *WET AND DRY*
If you have access to a heat source in the wilderness (such as a fire) and water, place the water in a receptacle and warm it until it is around 100 degrees (test the water with an unaffected part of your body to make sure it is warm, but not scalding). Immerse the frostbitten area into the water until it turns bright red. This won't feel great, to put it mildly, and your skin will likely break out into blisters thanks to the trauma of freezing and unfreezing blood vessels. Don't pop or break those blisters if possible. Gently dry the area and loosely wrap it with gauze or bandages to protect it from infection (but don't bind fingers or toes together in a single wad of bandages if they have been frostbitten—you want to keep all your little piggies separated).

3. *WAIT AND SEE*
You've now done all you can to treat the frostbite on your own and need to get to trained medical professionals as soon as possible. They can help manage the intense pain your damaged tissue is causing you and will observe you over the next 24 to 48 hours. If the damaged skin turns black, that's...not great. It means the frostbite killed much of the tissue and gangrene has possibly set in, meaning you may have to part with some very well-loved digits or appendages. But better to lose them than your life, right?

HOW TO EVADE CAPTURE IN THE WILDERNESS

VEN THE bravest and toughest among us may occasionally need to make themselves scarce and shake off a dogged pursuit in the wild. Maybe you're evading roving bands of cannibals after SHTF (Stuff Hits the Fan), or maybe you're just engaged in an epic game of hide-and-seek. Whatever the case, we'll teach you how to put in practice the old adage "Discretion is the better part of valor."

1. *GO THE DISTANCE*

A running head start won't shake anyone seriously trying to follow you, but it will give you more time to plan your next several moves. If you are aware someone is onto you, try and put as much distance between you and them as possible. They may be able to follow your steps, but you'll have bought yourself some time.

2. *ATTENTION TO DETAIL*

Once you're confident of the lead you have on your pursuers, you need to slow down in order to move in a manner that leaves as little of a trail as possible. You probably can't completely lose a competent tracker, but there's plenty you can do to mislead and slow them down. If practical, rip up extra clothing and use the pieces to wrap up your shoes, which minimizes your shoeprint and obscures the treadmark pattern. Step carefully and try to avoid breaking branches and twigs. Remember you are purposefully sacrificing speed for stealth, so don't panic because you aren't barrelling through the forest.

3. *MASTER MISDIRECTION*

In general, you should avoid roads, as your pursuers will most likely expect you to gravitate toward them. But you can also use paved trails or highways to turn the tables on your trackers. If you're feeling bold, travel up a little ways on a road and cross to the other side, purposefully leaving a trail of dirt, mud, broken branches, etc. for your trackers to follow. Venture into the woods or grass for a bit, and then double back to the road. Making sure the bottoms of your shoes are immaculate, walk down the opposite direction from your false trail, taking care not to leave any signs of your passage.

4. *GET DIRTY*

If you're wearing your favorite fluorescent thermal during your pursuit, that's going to draw the eye of any pursuers in the vicinity. The quickest and most effective form of camouflage lies all around you in the form of mud, which you should smear all over you. Not only will mud reduce the shine of your skin, it'll also help you blend in with the ground should you need to avoid being spotted by nearby trackers.

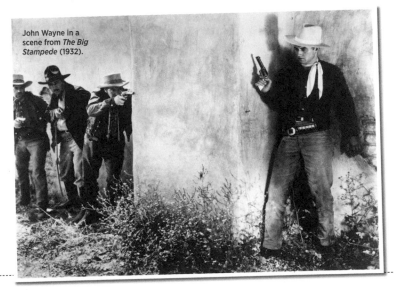

John Wayne in a scene from *The Big Stampede* (1932).

HOW TO SURVIVE AN AVALANCHE

 OU MIGHT EXACTLY AS WELL try to outrun a burst from a Lewis gun fired directly at your back as try to ski ahead of an avalanche. There is only one thing to do. Swim in it as though you were in the water and try and keep your head from being buried." While Ernest Hemingway's advice from his *Toronto Star Weekly* piece "Swiss Avalanches" wasn't necessarily complete, he was onto something almost 100 years ago as he learned to ski in the Austrian Alps. When an avalanche—essentially a landslide where snow is displaced instead of Earth—occurs, it is an immediate danger to most life on the mountain, and definitely to any humans. According to *National Geographic*, avalanches kill at least 150 people worldwide each year, most of whom are snowmobilers, skiiers or snowboarders. So if there's some winter activities in your future, knowing how to act during one of these rare but devastating incidents might just be life-saving.

1. *BEACON YOURSELF*

The first precaution you can take against being injured or killed in an avalanche is to take advantage of technology. If you're traveling with a partner—and you should be—a pair of transceivers can send a beacon between the two of you and allow one to find the other in case of

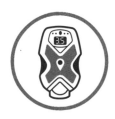

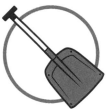

emergency. A more precise beacon known as an avalanche probe can help pinpoint someone in the aftermath. And a GPS locator coupled with simply letting people know where you'll be could mean the difference between life and death. It is also prudent to carry some kind of shovel with you. It might not be the most advanced tech, but a shovel digs more than five times faster than bare hands.

2. *MAKE A QUICK DECISION*
If caught in an avalanche, the first reaction you make should have a lot to do with what you're doing on the mountain in the first place. If you're on skis or a snowboard, start by going downhill, gain speed, then veer to the side to try getting off the moving snow. If you're hiking and the avalanche starts under your

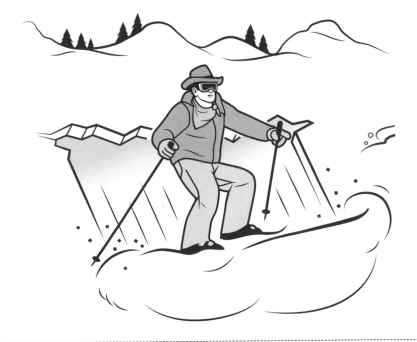

boots, try running uphill and to the side to get off of the fracturing pieces of snow. If you're on a snowmobile, don't change direction. Gun it and try to get off the fracturing piece of snow.

3. DO LIKE PAPA TOLD YOU

If it becomes clear that you're not going to beat the avalanche with speed and change of direction, drop your equipment and abandon your snowmobile. The goal is to be as light as possible and incorporate the "swimming" technique Hemingway mentioned. But simply trying to ride the snow like you would ride a wave to shore will likely end in disaster. Most of the debris being churned up by the avalanche is contained at the head of the wave, making your chances of injury much higher. Instead, roll onto your back with your feet downhill. Try to swim uphill doing the backstroke, which keeps your face out of the snow as much as possible.

4. IF YOU CAN, GRAB ON TO A TREE

Grab a tree and get as high as you can, advice that is much more useful at the beginning of an avalanche. Once one gets moving, it can reach 80mph, and grabbing a tree at 80mph is like grabbing the hood of a car going the same speed.

5. IF YOU ARE SUBMERGED

Approximately 25 percent of avalanche fatalities are due to blunt trauma, which technically makes those who survive to the end of an avalanche relatively lucky. But they are immediately faced with another split second in which their actions determine whether they live or die. Once the snow stops moving,

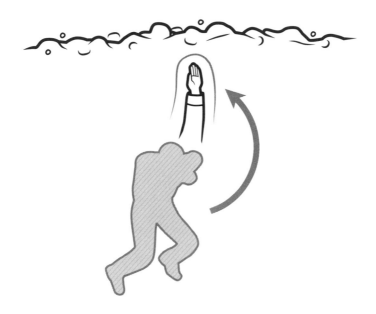

it will begin to set, refreezing into place. Put your arm across your face to create an air pocket and take a deep breath so your chest and stomach are puffed out. The goal is to give yourself as much breathing room as possible. If you're near the surface, try punching an arm or kicking a leg up through, which will make finding you much easier.

6. *STAY CALM*

It's not so easy when you're in the aftermath of an event like an avalanche, but it's important to remember that the more slowly you are able to breathe, the less oxygen you use and the more time you have to be rescued.

HOW TO KICK DOWN A DOOR

HEN IS A DOOR NOT A DOOR? When it's standing between you and where you need to be. Maybe there's a friend on the other side in urgent need of your help or maybe you just locked your keys in your home but you don't have the time or patience to pick the lock. Either way, you can use brute strength to force your way through.

1. *CHECK THE HINGES*

You have to make sure the door will be able to be kicked down. If the door opens away from you, then you're in luck! It's nearly impossible to kick down a door if it opens toward you. If you try, you'll only hurt your leg (and pride).

2. *GET INTO POSITION AND AIM*

Make sure you stand about a leg's length away— too close or far away, and you won't be able to use the full power of your kick. You also need to aim your kick wisely. The best place to make impact is at the door's weakest part—the area around the lock. Aim either right above it or right below it. Just don't kick the actual lock, or it will be your foot that shatters and not the door.

3. *NOW KICK!*

The time is now. Take your dominant leg and use a front kick to knock that door down. Drive your heel into the door. You're not a ballerina, so no need to use your toes. Use all your effort and emotions to knock down the door (again,

the context for why you're knocking this door down is between you, the door and what's on the other side).
Keep on repeating until the door is finally knocked down (or until you determine the door has won the battle).

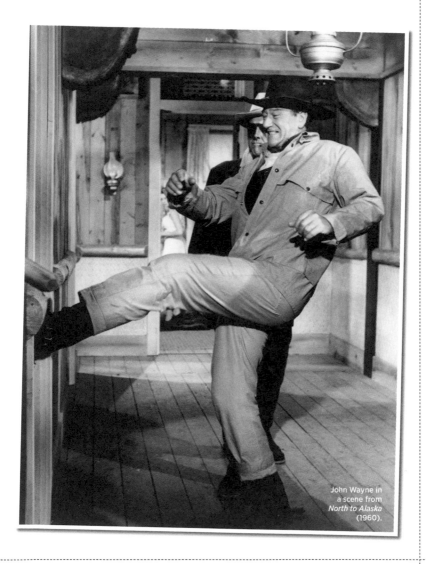

John Wayne in a scene from *North to Alaska* (1960).

HOW TO DRIVE DURING A FLASH FLOOD

 HEN WHAT STARTED OUT as a run-of-the-mill downpour has turned into a deluge from the skies implying someone, somewhere has begun gathering animals two by two in preparation for the storm, it's time to fully assess your ability to drive during flash flood conditions. Among the most dangerous and life-threatening weather disasters confronted by Americans, a flash flood can sweep your car into an overflowing river before you can dial for help. But there's no need to panic because the driving tips outlined here will help you make it to safety and survive to tell the tale about how you almost drowned.

1. *SLOW IT DOWN*

Some of the biggest dangers you face in attempting to drive through a flooded road are taking water in the engine (which will leave you stranded and at the mercy of the sweeping current) and losing control of the vehicle, both of which increase as your speedometer rises. Take it slow to avoid hydroplaning (where the water between the tire and the ground makes you spin out of control) and to help prevent water from sloshing in your engine.

2. *GIVE IN TO PEER PRESSURE*

It's difficult to judge the depth of water on the road. Flooded roads can be murky, and potholes can be impossible to detect. Be on the lookout for other cars on the road, and base your judgements on their driving. Did they make a big splash? Was there a deep pothole? This can help you estimate how deep the water ahead of you actually is.

3. *WATCH OUT*
Avoid anything floating in the water, especially downed power lines. Driving through electrified water is a huge no-no, particularly if circumstances force you to evacuate the vehicle. Keep calm, and steer yourself to dry land and safety.

HOW TO WALK THROUGH A FLOOD

What's worse than being caught in your car during a flash flood? Having to face the flood when there's nothing between you and the raging waters. While most of the survival tips here fall firmly under the header of common sense, it's still good to brush up on the basics.

1. Head for higher ground. Not home. Not back to your car. Finding higher ground above the waters is your one and only priority. Once you manage to get to someplace safe, stay there until help arrives.

2. Avoid water at all costs. Even if the water looks shallow and placid, keep in mind it only takes about six inches of moving water to knock you on your keister and potentially carry you to someplace less safe.

3. If you have to cross water, use a stick to try and test its depth. Make sure the ground underneath is solid and not slick mud. And if you do get knocked down and swept up in the flood, grab something to hold on to as soon as you can. But then, you didn't need this book to tell you that, did you?

HOW TO ESCAPE A SINKING CAR

OU MAY SEE YOUR CAR or truck as the primary means to unprecedented personal freedom on the open road, but a vehicle submerged in the water is little more than a weighted death trap. Every year approximately 400 drivers in North America perish in a watery tomb, mostly due to panic clouding their thinking. Keeping a cool head and knowing what to do when the time comes can save your life (and the lives of anyone who picked the wrong day to hitch a ride with you).

1. *LET LOOSE*

Once you've made contact with the water, your car is likely to float for about 30 seconds. Stay calm and undo your safety belt (which has now become an un-safety belt).

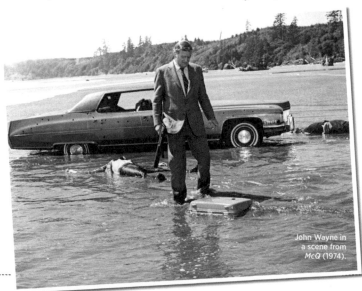

John Wayne in a scene from *McQ* (1974).

2. REACH YOUR BREAKING POINT

Although it may seem natural to try to leave through your car door, this is actually the least practical move to make. The surrounding water pressure will put a total of 600 pounds per square inch on your door, making it nearly impossible for you to open. This pressure will only disappear once the car has been completely filled with water, something you really don't want to experience. Opening the door will let in such an enormous amount of water the car will sink in seconds, making escape less likely. This makes your window the ideal escape point, especially because your car's electricity should stay on for at least three minutes, giving you ample time to get it open. Don't worry about water getting in through the window; that's the least of your worries right now as your main goal should be to escape. If your electricity is disabled, use a sharp object to break open the window. Don't try to break open the windshield because they are typically several layers thick.

3. SWIM FOR FREEDOM

Even with water pouring into your vehicle, you need to keep your wits about you and act quickly. Take a few very deep breaths until the water is up to your chin and then try to exit through the window. This will be much easier said than done since the water rushing through will make pushing out of it difficult. Still, it's much smarter to leave now than it is to wait for your car to sink farther down.

4. RISE TO THE CHALLENGE

Once you've exited the car, hold yourself in a tight position so that you'll naturally buoy yourself to the surface (now would be a great time to use the techniques found on page 62). Take a minute to orient yourself and identify what direction you should swim to reach safety. Then call your insurance guy.

HOW TO SET A BROKEN BONE

 NE SHOULD ALWAYS GO into the wilderness prepared for all eventualities, but that doesn't mean accidents won't happen. A broken bone out in the wild could result in serious injury—even death—if mishandled. A lack of resources can lead to permanent harm, and conditions such as shock can kill even after someone is properly splinted. Read on to discover what you can do to help a friend if things go south.

1. *EVALUATE THE SITUATION*
For starters, if the victim has a compound fracture (a break where the bone has punctured through the skin) you're going to need more than a splint. Get medical help immediately. Secondly, don't attempt to splint a neck or back injury, as the safest thing you can do if injuries to the spinal cord are suspected is to keep the victim completely still. If you're dealing with a less severe break, your next step should be finding someplace safe where you can tend to the wound in peace.

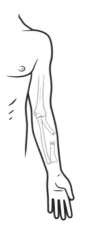

2. *KEEP THE FRACTURE STABLE*
One of the reasons a broken bone is so dangerous is that it can do serious harm to the surrounding tissue, nerves and blood vessels if not quickly stabilized. First, focus on minimizing the injured limb's movements. If professional medical attention is nearby, splint the fracture as is, and let a doctor handle the repairs. But if medical attention is hours (or days) away, grip the limb above the break (i.e. on the end of the limb closest to the body) with one hand to hold

it in place. With your other hand, grasp the limb below the break and gently apply downward pressure until the bones move back into place, then splint the limb as outlined in Step 3. This process won't feel great for your friend, and if they determine the movement makes the break feel more painful, release the pressure and splint the limb as is.

3. CREATE A SPLINT

Since you're out in the wilderness you're going to have to get creative with your splint. First grab two thick sticks that are about the size and length of the injured bone. Next find something you can use to tie them together, such as strips of cloth or even a belt. Place whatever you're using to tie the splint on the ground beneath the injured limb. Do not place the tie directly on the wound; instead you'll want to place the ties above and/or below the break. Take the sticks and place

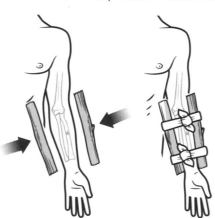

them on both sides of the injured limb, directly above the tying device. Take both ends of your tying material and secure them with a knot, so that the sticks are secure in their placement against the injured limb. Make sure the splint is stable but not so tight that it will halt circulation.

4. CHECK FOR SHOCK

Shock can kill even if the injury is properly splinted. Signs of shock include a fluttering heartbeat, clammy skin, a confused mental state and a blue complexion. If the victim shows signs of shock keep them warm at all costs. Place them in a comfortable position and cover them in a blanket or even a pile of leaves. Also, make sure to keep the victim hydrated to help combat the effects of shock.

HOW TO STOP MAJOR BLEEDING

OST OF THE TIME you accidently draw blood, whether nicking yourself shaving or being careless with a pair of scissors, you can staunch the wound with a simple bandage. That is not the kind of bleeding discussed here. You're reading this because you want to know how to deal with the kind of wound that turns your surroundings into something resembling the lobby of the Overlook Hotel. The human body contains roughly 9–12 pints of blood, and you can spill about half of that before it's game over. Your obvious goal should be to seek professional medical attention, but the advice below should help you staunch the wound so you can get there.

1. *DON'T PULL IT OUT*
If the source of your woe started when you were impaled with a sharp object (rock, stick, sword, etc.) whatever you do, don't pull it out. The presence of the object is likely preventing even more blood from exiting, which means you want to leave it in there.

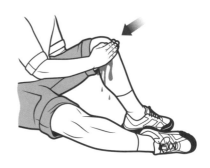

2. *KEEP UP THE PRESSURE*
Boiled down, your conundrum is that life-sustaining blood is trying to leave your body through a hole or gap. You want it to stay put. Your first order of business is putting sustained

pressure on the wound, preferably with a clean bandage, but a torn up piece of clothing (such as a T-shirt) will also suffice.

3. *KICK UP YOUR BOOTS*
One of the biggest dangers of a major wound is losing so much blood that your heart, starved of oxygen, stops acting as an efficient pump. Called hypovolemic shock, this condition leads to major organ failure, which is not a good look for you. One way to help combat shock is to lie down with your feet elevated above your chest, if possible. If you've suffered a neck, head or back injury, though, you shouldn't move at all.

4. *TIE IT TOGETHER*
If the blood pumps out of your wound with the same rhythm as your heartbeat, that means you've severed an artery and need to take more drastic action than simple pressure to staunch the flow of blood. You need a tourniquet. Take a belt or torn piece of clothing and tie it tightly a few inches above the wound on your limb (if the wound is on your abdomen or neck, the tourniquet won't work). You've successfully cut off the flow of blood to the wound, but that also means you stopped blood flowing to the entire limb. It takes at least two hours of wearing the torniquet before the muscles start getting damaged, and up to six hours before amputation becomes probable. So get yourself some professional medical attention ASAP. That said, you'd much rather have a prosthetic leg and a story to tell than to reach your end in a puddle of your own blood, right?

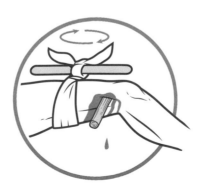

HOW TO UNTIE A TOUGH KNOT

HETHER ATTEMPTING TO FREE a damsel in distress tied to a railroad track or trying to free your foot from an ornery bootlace, you need to know the ins and outs of loosening knots so you can easily untie one in a pinch.

1. DO THE TWIST

Start twisting one loose end of the knot as tight as you can. Your goal is to turn this loose end into something as compact and rigid as possible. This will lessen the friction holding the knot together and create some slack. Once you get it really tight, start pushing the twisted portion into the knot—it should slide through easily.

2. JUST TAP IT

Another way to loosen the knot is by giving it a couple of hard taps against a hard surface. The force of your assault should help relax the knot into something easier to untie, so don't feel the need to hold back.

3. USE YOUR TOOLS

If you have a bobby pin or some tweezers lying around, either of those tools could help you loosen up your knot. Poke your tool through the knot to break up the tight bond and then untie it on your own.

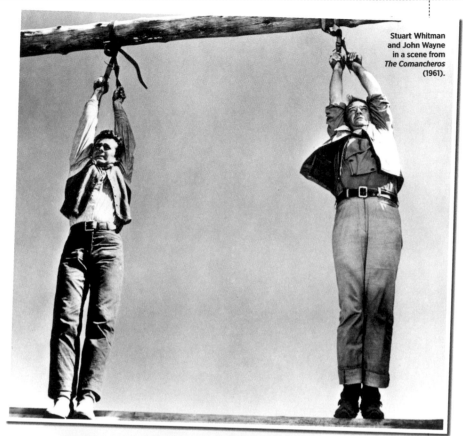

Stuart Whitman
and John Wayne
in a scene from
The Comancheros
(1961).

HOW TO SLIP YOUR BONDS

Most of us will (hopefully) go through life without having our hands bound against our will. But on the off chance you do find yourself all tied up, here's how you can free your hands.

1. Rotate your wrists back and forth repeatedly. It may take a while, but the bond should loosen and you can slip free of the rope.

2. If your captor used a zip tie, your goal is to break the tie where it locks. If possible, lift your bound hands over your head and then quickly bring them down into your abdomen while simultaneously trying to pull your wrists apart. Repeat this motion until you've managed to break the locks and set yourself free.

HOW TO SURVIVE FALLING INTO ICY WATER

ON'T LET A plunge into the cold wet be the afternoon dip that ends your life. Keep calm, follow the advice below and give yourself a fighting chance.

1. *DON'T BREATHE*

As soon as your body hits the freezing water, you're going to enter what experts call "cold shock." Adrenaline shoots through your body and your heart rate skyrockets, just two of the immediate physiological changes that cause you to have a hyperventilation reflex. For obvious reasons, you want to fight these reflexes with all your might and get your head above water as soon as possible. It takes roughly 1-3 minutes before your body acclimates (somewhat) to the dangerous temperature it finds itself in.

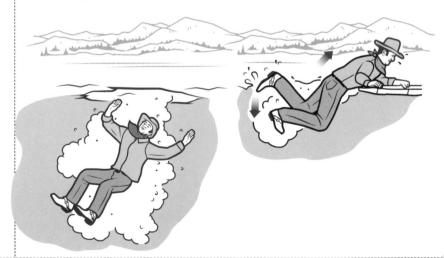

2. *GET OUT*

You're now in the deadliest race of your life against the cold's debilitating effects on muscle coordination and movement. You probably have at most five minutes after plunging into the water before you can no longer swim yourself to safety. Your priority is to locate and swim to the hole you fell through, as that's your most reliable point of exit from what can potentially become your icy grave. Once you locate the hole, put as much of your upper body as possible on the surface, then repeatedly kick your legs (while pushing/ pulling yourself up with your arms) to get your entire body out of the water.

3. *ROLL WITH IT*

You've made it out of the water, but not out of danger. Your main foe is now your dropping core body temperature, which can still kill you. To minimize the risk of falling through the ice again, roll away from the opening and toward warm, dry shelter—preferably a vehicle or a tent, but even a rock or tree can do.

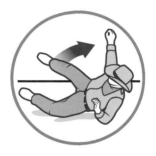

4. *STRIP AND SIZZLE*

Congratulations! You didn't drown. But hypothermia could still claim your life, and your soaked clothes will prevent any sources of heat from warming you up efficiently. Strip them off. Tuck your knees up to your chest and cross your arms across your chest to conserve heat. You'll also want to find dry clothes and an external heat source (a fire or a car's heater) as soon as you're able. (For more on how to keep your body temperature up, see page 56.)

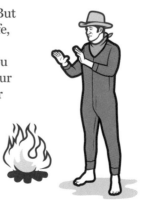

HOW TO GET THE POWER BACK ON

 OBODY ENJOYS the frustration of a sudden power outage ruining a night of watching John Wayne movies (or whatever else people depend on electricity for). But a blackout does give you the chance to demonstrate your handy skills by restoring the power. Grab the flashlight or candles and matches you have stored for emergencies like this one and follow the tips below—you'll have the lights back on in no time.

1. *GO TO THE SOURCE*
If you're living somewhere that's just weathered a lightning storm, hurricane or Godzilla rampage, you can bet the problem with your power lies with your provider. But if the lights went off for no apparent reason, and it appears your neighbors still have their lights on, you should find your circuit breaker or fuse box—your home will have one or the other. The usual places to find it include the garage, a storeroom, basement or even outside. You're looking for a metal box protected by a cover. Once you find the box, open it up and see what you're dealing with.

2. *WHATCHA GOT?*
If your house has a circuit breaker, you'll see a box with a row of switches. If it's a fuse box,

you'll be staring at a row of...wait for it...fuses. These look kind of like small light bulbs. In either case, make sure the lights are switched off and all major appliances in the house are unplugged before you start fiddling with the insides of the box. And if you have a fuse box, wear a pair of rubber gloves just to be safe.

3. *SCREW IT (OR FLIP IT)*
Those dealing with a fuse box will need to check which fuse has blown. Turn off the main power using the switch almost certainly located near the top of the inside of the box, and get ready for some repair work. Check each fuse for discoloration or if it has a bit of melted metal inside it—that's the blown fuse. Unscrew and replace with a fresh one you can pick up at any hardware store (just make sure the new fuse is of the same amperage as the replacement). Flip the main power back on and close up the box. If you have a circuit breaker, look to see which of the switches is out of line with the others. Flip that switch all the way off and then back to its proper position.

3. *BACK IN BUSINESS*
Now test out whether your mission was successful by flipping on the lights. If you are bathed in the glow of electricity (and self-satisfaction), you know you nailed it.

HOW TO HOTWIRE A CAR

BEING A RUGGED INDIVIDUALIST means, in the best John Wayne tradition, you also respect the rights and property of others. However, in certain extreme survival situations, you need to make the choice between following the letter of the law and preserving your life. Being placed in such a conundrum is the only acceptable excuse to hotwire a stranger's car.

First off, you need to understand that most vehicles made since about 2000 are exponentially more difficult to hotwire than those made in the Before Times, requiring specialized equipment and technical knowledge of specific models you're unlikely to have in a survival situation. Hopefully the car you need to start is old.

1. *MAKE AN ENTRANCE*

If you do come across a car or truck dating from the Clinton administration or earlier, your first order of business is to gain access to the vehicle's interior. Unless you've gotten stranded on a return trip to the

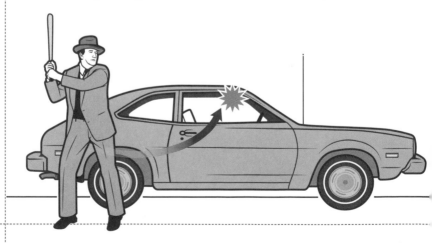

dry cleaners, you probably don't have a coat hanger on hand to help you open the door. But that's OK because you do possess the brute strength needed to safely shatter the window. Take a sharp object (ideally a screwdriver or the claw end of a hammer, but even an edged rock would do) and strike it with force at the edge of the window pane—where the glass is weakest. It should shatter into tiny pieces, giving you easy access to the car's lock on the inside.

2. *GET WIRED*

When you are hotwiring a car, your goal is to connect the power from the car's battery with the ignition/electric systems and the starter, a process you normally initiate every time you turn the ignition lock with your key. You need to bypass that ignition lock by accessing the wires in the steering column directly and connecting the proper wires by hand. To get a hold of the wires, look under the steering column for a plastic panel—it may be screwed into the column, but you should be able to force it open if necessary to reveal a huge bundle of wires.

It may look like complete chaos, but a closer examination should reveal the wires are grouped in three major bundles. Two of the bundles should lead to either side of the car, as they control the dashboard lights, blinkers, electric seat adjusters, etc. But one bundle should run straight up into the steering column, and that's the one you'll be working with.

3. *BRING IT TOGETHER*

The bundle of wires you need to focus on should be comprised of at least three wires, each a different color. You're trying to identify the wire for the battery, the wire for the ignition and the starter wire. The wire for the battery is usually red no matter what model of vehicle, but the colors for the other two can vary. Through trial and error, you'll have to figure out which

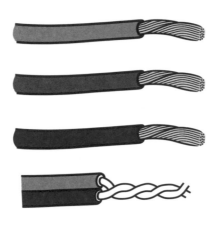

wire connects to which system.

Take the battery wire and the ignition wire and, using a sharp object, carefully cut away the insulation from the ends of both wires (about an inch will do). If you have any electrical tape on hand, bind the ends of both these wires together, but if not, twist the ends of the wires so they connect. The lights and power for the car's interior should now be activated.

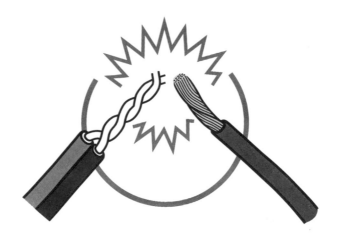

4. *START ME UP*

Now take the starter wire and CAREFULLY strip it of its insulation with your sharp object—remember that this is now a live wire. To start the engine, take the end of this wire and tap it on the end of the ignition/battery wires you bundled together, which should create a spark. Once the engine starts, rev it up a few times to prevent it from stalling, and you're almost good to go. Just make sure you bind the wires to the side with a ripped piece of clothing, tape, etc., so you don't accidently zap yourself when driving. You also need to break the lock on the steering wheel, but that's as simple as turning the wheel hard to one direction, keeping sustained pressure on the lock until it snaps. Now drive yourself to safety and make sure to leave a nice "thanks for the ride, sorry for the mess"-style note on the windshield after you're done with it.

HOW TO SURVIVE A LIGHTNING STORM OUTDOORS

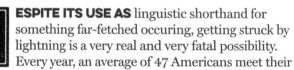

ESPITE ITS USE AS linguistic shorthand for something far-fetched occuring, getting struck by lightning is a very real and very fatal possibility. Every year, an average of 47 Americans meet their end via a 5,000-degree bolt of electricity, and men are four times more likely to be struck than women. Here's how to put the odds further in your favor.

1. *GET LOW*

If you're caught outside during a lightning storm and can't find a safe shelter (please note your tent doesn't qualify) then you need to get busy finding the lowest spot possible in your area. Lightning will always strike the highest available point, so avoid hilltops, solitary trees and abandoned windmills. Try to make it below the tree line so that a lush forest of giant, wooden targets is between you and the wrath of the heavens. You should also avoid caves, as the rock can sometimes be an excellent conductor of electricity from any nearby lightning strikes.

2. *LET GO*

If a lightning storm is approaching, relieve yourself of any metal objects on your person. Backpacks with metal frames, jewelry, the lightning rod you always carry around with you…it all needs to be left behind to collect after the storm passes.

3. SPREAD OUT

As callous as this step may seem, you want to make sure you're at least 50 feet away from anyone else during a lightning storm. Why? The human body does a great job conducting electricity, so you want to avoid getting caught in a chain reaction of disablement and death if one of your hiking buddies wins the world's unluckiest lottery. Think of it this way—you can't help (or plan a funeral for) your friend if you're in trouble yourself.

4. ASSUME THE POSITION

When you feel you've arrived at the safest position possible, maximize your chances of survival by minimizing the surface area of the ground in contact with your body. Crouch down on the balls of your feet, covering your ears with your hands to avoid damaging your hearing from the thunderclap. The thunder will be loud, and your howls may be louder.

HOW TO FIRE A FLARE GUN

HILE WE DON'T DOUBT your ability to handle most of life's problems, there are times when it's better to call for help. For those moments when you're trapped on a sinking ship or lost in the forest with no trail in sight, a flare gun can help you get back in contact with civilization. Knowing how to operate one correctly can help you avoid a trip to the hospital once they find you.

1. *GET UPWIND*
Position yourself so the wind is at your back. The slag and sparks released by a fired flare gun can easily end up on your face or arm if you ignore this step.

2. *KNOW YOUR HARDWARE*
Make sure you're familiar with the flare you're using. Some flares require you to pull off one cap, while others require two. Make sure it's loaded and that you're in a good position to fire.

3. *WEAR PROTECTION*
As previously mentioned, the discharge of a flare can do some damage if you're not careful. Always wear eye protection such as sunglasses or goggles so the bright light doesn't harm your eyes. Heat resistant gloves are just as useful since the barrel could heat up or the slag can drip down your arm. If you have none of the above, take precautions by wrapping your hand in a loose shirt and turning your head away when you fire.

4. *READY, AIM, FIRE!*
Hold the gun in your dominant hand and aim it at a 45-degree angle. Keep your arm straight and positioned

away from you. Flares burn extremely bright (which is why they can be seen for miles), so remember to look away when you fire to preserve your eyesight. If you're able, fire two flares in quick succession so authorities have an easier time locating you.

5. *CLEAN UP*
Get rid of the used flare shell by dropping it into water. This will make sure it doesn't cause an unexpected forest fire, the last thing you need if you're stuck on the side of a mountain.

HOW TO USE A SIGNAL MIRROR

Don't have a flare gun handy and can't be bothered to build a proper signal fire? You can still catch the attention of rescuers if you have a mirror or reflective piece of glass on your person. To do so, hold the mirror in your hand at eye level and angle it so it catches the sun's rays. Next, you want to hold your other arm at full-length and place that hand between the mirror and whoever you want to see your signal. The palm of your free hand should be facing you and you should spread your fingers apart enough so you can see the target (you're basically aiming where the light will go with this step). Once you have the light from the mirror hitting on your hand where you want it to, lower that free hand while keeping the mirror still. The bright light should now hit and attract the attention of the intended target.

HOW TO SURVIVE A TORNADO

 HERE ARE FEW THINGS more humbling than watching a tornado tear through a town. This unrepentant force of nature can flatten houses into the ground, and can do the same to anyone around it if they're not careful. A tornado can pick up cars, generate 300 mph winds and forever alter your feelings of safety. The best way to make sure you see the other side of the storm in one piece is to be prepared when one arrives.

1. *SCAN THE SKIES*
If you want to avoid suffering the wrath of a "finger of God," you first need to recognize when one is

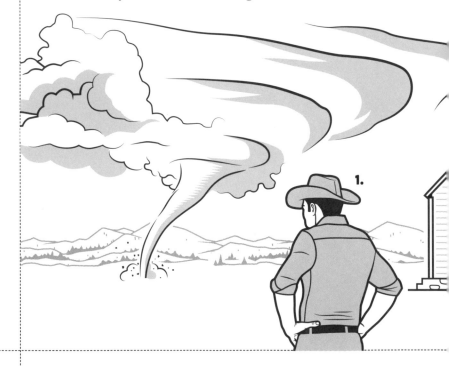

about to bear down on you. Look for the following types of storm clouds in the sky, which are strong indicators conditions are friendly for the formation of tornadoes:

- *Inflow Bands* Long, unbroken clouds extending out from the center of the storm that tell you the storm system is sucking up air from miles around— and if these clouds are curved or in a spiral, that means the air up there is likely to be rotating.

- *Beaver Tail* A smooth, single band of cloud sticking out from the main mass, this appendage also indicates rotation in the storm system.

- *Wall Cloud* An unbroken mass of cloud extended downward from the sky, this harbinger of havoc signals a tornado may be a mere 10 to 20 minutes away from forming.

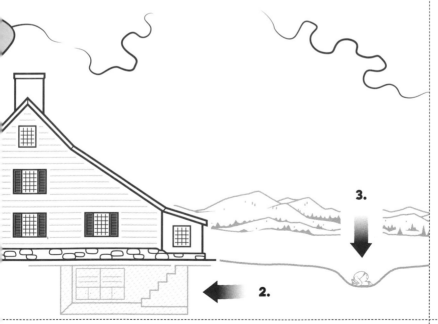

2. MAKE LIKE A MOLE

If you're indoors during a tornado warning, head underground immediately. If the building doesn't have a specifically prepared tornado shelter, a basement will work as well. The falling and flying debris created by a tornado is just as dangerous as the storm itself, so always make sure to cover yourself with a mattress or a table to prevent serious injury.

If you can't make it to a basement make sure to take some safety measures. Get away from high floors or rooms with a great deal of windows. Always take the stairs since an elevator can lose power. Mobile homes and long flat buildings are the most vulnerable to tornado damage and should be avoided at all costs.

3. LAY LOW

When caught in the open away from any obvious means of shelter, you have to do your best to stay covered and low to the ground. If you're in a car, never try to outdrive a tornado—if you see one near, stay put and do everything you can to take cover. Duck below the window and cover yourself with a coat or blanket in order to prevent any debris from making direct impact with your head. Facing a tornado in the wild without even a vehicle to protect you is the worst-case scenario, but you can still take action to maximize your chance for survival. Scan around for a ditch, a gully—any opportunity to get low. You may risk getting caught in flooding from rain, but the fact remains that staying in one place could help you avoid flying debris. Avoid hunkering down under an overpass on the highway. It's a common myth that an overpass is a safe place to take shelter, but they are vulnerable to structural damage, meaning chunks of steel and concrete could easily rain down on your head.

HOW TO SURVIVE AN EARTHQUAKE

Living most of his life in California, you can bet John Wayne knew what to do when the ground beneath his feet began trembling. Here are some basic steps to take if you find yourself caught in the middle of an earthquake.

1. Drop to your hands and knees. Chances are the earthquake is going to rock your world, and it is far better to get low in a gentle, controlled manner rather than to fall violently to the ground.

2. Crawl away from any windows and under something you know is sturdy (like that massive table you know won't collapse on you). Cover your head and neck with your arms to protect your most vulnerable areas.

3. If you are outside when the earthquake starts, move quickly away from any buildings, utility wires or streetlights. This may be easier said than done, but get out in the open as much as you can, then crouch down on your hands and knees as you would when indoors.

HOW TO BUILD A SIGNAL FIRE

 FIRE'S GOOD FOR MORE than just keeping you warm in the wilderness (though that's pretty important). With the proper techniques, you can create a controlled blaze that helps alert search and rescue teams to your presence. Here's how to make a fire nobody can ignore.

1. *BUILD HIGH*
There's no point trying to attract attention with a fire built in the inside of a cave hidden at the bottom of a valley. Instead, select an elevated site for your fire, such as the top of a hill. Just remember the principles of building a signal fire remain the same as any other flame, so you want to find a flat, dry spot with easy access to fuel.

2. *SMOKE 'EM IF YOU GOT 'EM*
More important than the flame itself will be the smoke your fire generates, and building a quick-and-easy tripod tower over your fire can help tremendously in that regard. Start by setting up your fire but don't ignite it. Then find three long sticks or branches (the longer the better) and position them in a tripod over the fire site, lashing the sticks together at the top with rope, your belt or something similar. Now find branches with plenty of green leaves on them and tie them to the branches of the tripod, leaving an opening so you can light the fire underneath. The result is a fire that's protected from the elements and will make plenty of smoke, thanks to the green leaves it will slowly consume.

3. *IF YOU CAN'T EAT IT, BURN IT*

Keep in mind the goal is to produce large volumes of thick, dark smoke that's easy to spot, so you'll want to find material that's not naturally combustible, which is more helpful than dead, dry twigs. Any man-made material you don't need such as plastic bags should go into the fire, as well as green plants. Smoke is just the result of fuel that can't be completely consumed by the flame, so the harder it is to burn, the better. Just don't overload the blaze so much you accidentally snuff it out.

HOW TO SAVE SOMEONE FROM DROWNING

ROM POOL PARTIES to days on the beach and beyond, water is both necessary for survival as well as a source of endless entertainment. It can also prove deadly, with almost 4,000 Americans accidentally drowning each year. If you happen to

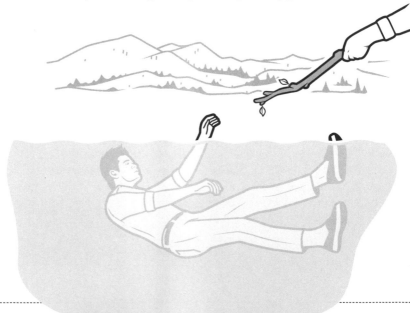

spot someone who looks like they are going to become a statistic, remember the information you'll learn here and help save the day.

1. ***STAY OUT OF THE WATER (IF YOU CAN)***
When you spot someone you suspect is in danger of drowning, repress your heroic, John Wayne-sized instincts to rush into the water and drag the victim to safety. You could just as easily end up joining the hapless swimmer in a fight for your life. A drowning person is one whose fight-or-flight response has completely taken over, meaning the victim can easily cling, kick or incapacitate you during your would-be rescue. If the person in need of help is close enough to shore (or the side of a pool, a boat, etc.) extend an object such as an oar, a branch, a towel, a lawn chair...anything the victim can grasp. Then pull the person to safety.

2. ***SWIM TO SAFETY***
If the victim is too far from land or safety for you to reach, you'll have to bring yourself closer to them. Again, avoid getting too close to the victim—while you're trying to rescue the person in distress, you need to treat him or her like a danger in order to pull off the rescue. Quickly strip off any heavy clothing and swim out to the drowning person, taking with you something to extend their way— ideally a life preserver ring, but more likely a towel or shirt. Swim near to the person (but not too near) and extend the object to the victim. When they grab it, swim in a straight direction back to safety with the person in tow, checking behind you every few minutes to make sure they're still holding on.

3. *CHECK FOR VITALS*

Once you've gotten the victim to shore, you need to make sure your hard work wasn't for naught. Check to see if they are breathing, and if that test comes up negative, check their pulse for 10 seconds by placing your index and middle finger against the underside of the wrist or the side of the neck. If no vitals are present, you should call 911 and perform CPR.

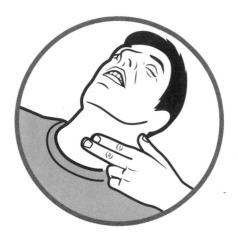

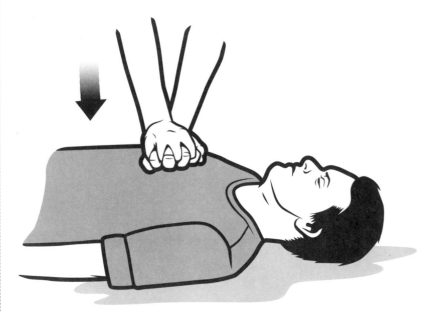

HOW TO AVOID DROWNING ON DRY LAND

Say what? Yup, you can still drown on dry land, and we don't mean from falling asleep in a bowl of soup. After being saved from a near-drowning experience, some suffer the misfortune of having their airways close up due to spasms caused by the presence of water still sloshing around where it shouldn't be. This can happen hours after the rescue, turning a lucky save into a tragedy.

When you've pulled someone out of the water (or are pulled out yourself), look out for these signs.

1. Persistent coughing and wheezing

2. Irritability, lethargy or general confusion caused by a slow deprivation of oxygen.

3. Chest pain. Dry drowning isn't very common, but it is a real phenomenon. It's also the main reason that, no matter what, you should always seek medical attention after a close call with drowning, regardless of how safe you seem.

HOW TO ESCAPE A RIPTIDE

HAT'S THE MOST dangerous killer stalking America's beaches? If you answered sharks, think again. It's actually riptides, the silent, invisible stalker of the ocean waiting to drag swimmers out to Davy Jones's Locker. More than 100 Americans are killed by riptides every year, mostly due to not knowing how to fight one. Riptides are incredibly strong currents that can pull even the strongest swimmers far out to sea. The key to escaping one involves going against some of your body's natural reactions to harm, so pay careful attention to the following advice.

1. *GO WITH THE FLOW*
   Once you've identified you are caught in a riptide do not fight against it. Although it goes against all of our instincts, fighting a riptide will only tire you out while doing little to help you escape. Riptides pull at a rate of eight feet per second, which puts swimming to safety out of the question. Try to stay calm and remember that a riptide can't pull you underwater, only farther out to sea.

2. *PARALLEL IS PERFECT*
   As counterproductive as it might seem, your best bet when it comes to escaping a rip current is to begin swimming parallel to the shore. Although currents are very strong, they're also very narrow, making escape a possibility. Calmly but purposefully swim parallel to the shore and don't panic if it still pulls you out to the ocean a little; you can easily get back to shore once you've escaped it. If you've conserved your energy by

not fighting the current, you shouldn't have an issue getting back to dry land.

3. *BACK TO THE BEACH*
Once the current is no longer pulling you, it's relatively easy to get back to safety. Swimming diagonally to the shore will ensure that you do not become caught in the current once again.

HOW TO SURVIVE A TSUNAMI

Now you know how to survive a treacherous tide that catches you in the water. But what do you do when the tide comes to find you on land? A tsunami is obviously a threat on a whole different level of magnitude than a riptide, but one that you may have to contend with if you reside in a coastal area prone to them.

1. The first thing to do is keep a vigilant eye on news reports about a possible tsunami in your area. That doesn't mean calling the local weatherman every day asking, "Hey, will there be a tsunami today?" But if experts detect an earthquake in the middle of the ocean (a possible indicator that a killer wave is on its way), then you can be sure they'll get the message out, so keep your eyes and ears open.

2. Evacuate the area. This doesn't mean head up the nearest hill, but rather a total evacuation to someplace the authorities are saying is safe.

3. If evacuation is impossible for whatever reason (and not wanting to leave your home is not a good reason), climb to the top of a three-story or higher building and hope for the best.

HOW TO EXTRACT A CAR STUCK IN SNOW, MUD OR ALMOST ANYTHING ELSE

S AN AMERICAN, the call of the open road is in your blood, beckoning you to find your next adventure down that long stretch of highway. Which is why getting stuck in the snow, ice or mud is particularly infuriating, impeding your God-given right to get where you need to be. Don't lose your cool the next time you find your wheels spinning—follow these tips and you'll be back on the road in no time.

1. *DO A WALKAROUND*
The first thing you need to do won't help you get unstuck, but it could save your life. Check your vehicle's tailpipe to ensure it isn't clogged with snow, mud or whatever, which could cause deadly carbon monoxide to build up in your vehicle and potentially kill you.

2. *CAN YOU DIG IT?*
Gunning the gas pedal will only cause your wheels to spin and dig the vehicle deeper into the hole you've made for yourself. Instead, take a shovel (or other digging tool) and clear out the snow or mud from around the tires. The 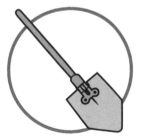 goal is to create an area where the tires can gain traction and get you unstuck. If you have anything to help your tires get traction (kitty litter, car mats, a towel, etc.), place it in front of your tires before attempting to drive again.

3. *BACK AND FORTH*

Get inside your vehicle and start the engine. Turn the steering wheel so your tires are as straight as possible, and then back up slowly, stop, and then drive forward just as carefully (you don't want to rev the engine and ruin the transmission). Repeat this technique until you build up enough traction to become unstuck.

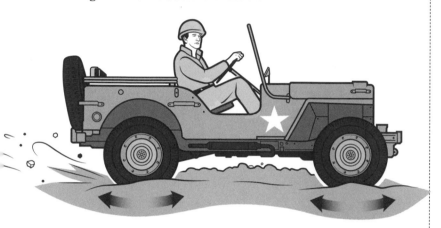

4. *LET OUT SOME AIR*

A method you should only use as a last resort, letting some air out of your tires increases the amount of rubber making contact with the ground, which also ups the amount of traction you gain. However, you need to make sure you'll be able to refill those tires quickly after you break free, as driving on deflated ones can seriously damage your wheels.

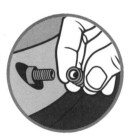

5. *GET OUT*

Once you manage to get unstuck, don't let off the gas. You want to keep the momentum going until you are sure you're clear of the treacherous ground, otherwise you risk getting stuck all over again.

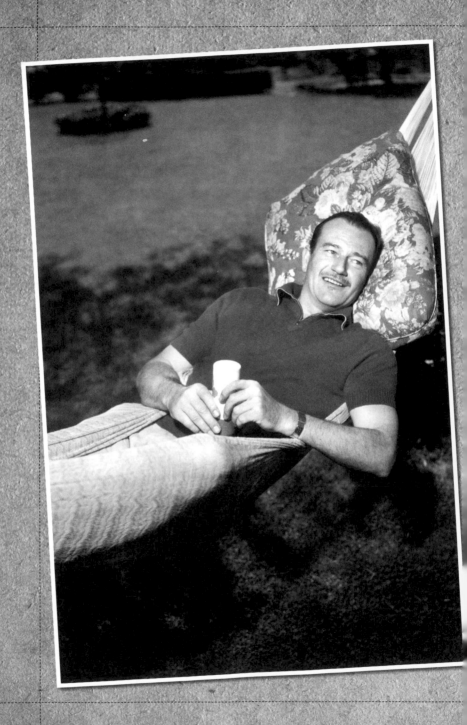

AT HOME

BEING HANDY AROUND
THE HOUSE CAN
BE ONE OF MAN'S
GREATEST PLEASURES

HOW TO BE YOUR DOG'S ALPHA

ITHOUT QUESTION, dogs are man's best friend. But if you don't take the proper precautions, your canine companion will be the kind of friend who crashes on your couch for a month, eats all of your food and makes a mess of the bathroom. Like their distant wolf cousins, dogs are looking for someone to tell them what to do. They need a leader and you need to step up to the plate or else they will. With these four tips, you can get a good start on turning your pooch into a pal for life.

1. *STRAIGHTEN UP*

Your dog takes note of your body language when you give commands. Make sure you're standing up straight and keep your hands out of your pockets. If you're sitting down when you give a command, your dog might not take you seriously. When your dog masters "sit and stay" in one room, make sure to move around to the other areas of the house, so they recognize you have authority in every room.

2. *PILE ON THE PRAISE*

As far as your dog is concerned, you're speaking a foreign language. When they correctly interpret that you want them to lay down, you should respond verbally with "Yes" or use a clicker to mark their behavior, along with a treat for praise, so they associate that sound or word with the proper response.

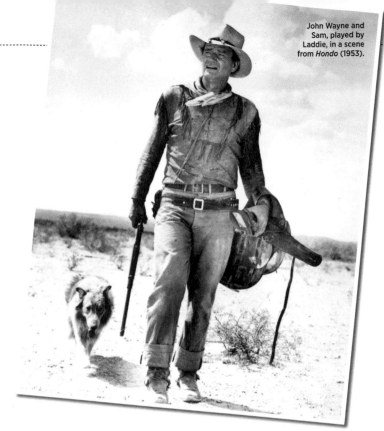

John Wayne and Sam, played by Laddie, in a scene from *Hondo* (1953).

3. *BUT NOT TOO MUCH*

Remember that your pooch is pretty smart. If you have a bag of treats in your hand while you're teaching them commands, they'll listen to you. But when that bag is gone, they don't have any incentive to comply. Use treats sparingly and only let your dog know that you have treats after they've completed your command successfully. The key to success is to be consistent.

4. *KEEP 'EM OCCUPIED!*

Sure, dogs could eat treats all day if you'd let them, but they also love a long walk or playing fetch in the yard. After your dog behaves the way you've taught them to, reward them with a trip to the dog park, a springy new tennis ball or a big-time belly rub.

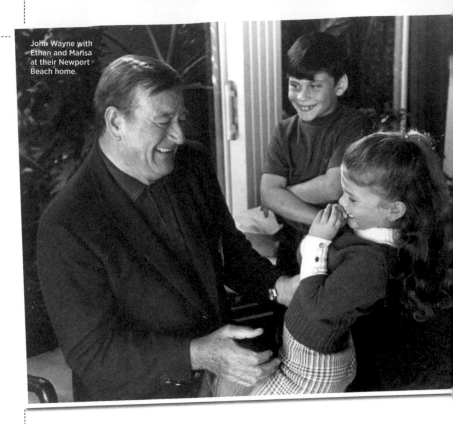

John Wayne with Ethan and Marisa at their Newport Beach home.

HOW TO RAISE 'EM RIGHT

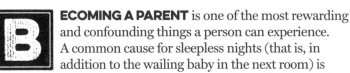

BECOMING A PARENT is one of the most rewarding and confounding things a person can experience. A common cause for sleepless nights (that is, in addition to the wailing baby in the next room) is obsessing over the question "How am I screwing this kid up?" The bad news is that you probably can't avoid some mishaps— no one's perfect. Duke often engaged in tough love with his children, but the emphasis was always on love. Try teaching your kids these three lessons the Wayne children learned well.

1. *TEACH THEM TO BE RESPECTFUL*

It's a tough lesson that we all need to learn at some point, and Marisa Wayne, Duke's youngest daughter, learned this one the hard way. When she let her room on the *Wild Goose* get messy, her father asked her to pick up her clothes. After Marisa ignored her father's request, Duke began throwing her clothes overboard. According to Marisa, "It all came down to disrespect, and in his mind it was disrespectful that I wasn't picking up after myself."

2. *TEACH THE VALUE OF HARD WORK*

Anyone who knows anything about Duke knows he found success by working for it. He passed these same values on to his children, as Patrick Wayne knows well. When his horsemanship wasn't up to par while filming *The Comancheros* (1961), his father admonished him, stating, "You're going to learn how to ride now or get out of the business." And learn he did: Patrick worked to improve his riding, and soon he could ride as well as any cowboy, just like his father.

3. *TEACH THEM TO BE RESPONSIBLE*

Your child can't grow into a kind, responsible adult if he or she isn't given any responsibilities. Setting up a consistent schedule of chores helps teach your child the value of managing time, as well as a lesson about meeting expectations. This was one of the tools Duke used to teach his own children some responsibility. As his son Ethan remembers: "I think he did a lot of things that created responsibility for a young person. There were chores everyday. If you were on the boat, there were chores. If you were on location, there were chores. If you wanted to ride a horse, you had to take care of it. You had to assume all the responsibilities: feed it, clean it, brush it, saddle it, etc."

HOW TO
CHANGE A TIRE

EMEMBER THAT SCENE where John Wayne gets a flat tire and calls AAA? No? That's because rugged individualists like Duke need a AAA card about as much as a fish needs roller blades. The next time you get a flat, roll up your sleeves and call the best person for the job—yourself.

1. *KEEP 'ER STEADY*

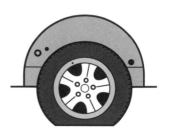

Before you do anything, make sure you've stopped your vehicle in a flat, level area. Trying to change a tire anywhere else can easily lead to your vehicle rolling off on its own, causing all sorts of mayhem. If it can be avoided, don't change the tire on the side of the road or highway, as this exposes you to oncoming traffic. Also, while it should go without saying, make sure you've placed the car in park and engaged the emergency brake.

2. *NICE AND LOOSE*

Take out the spare tire, jack and lug wrench you always keep in your vehicle because you are the kind of prepared individual who plans for the worst. Take the wrench and loosen the lug nuts on the wheel with

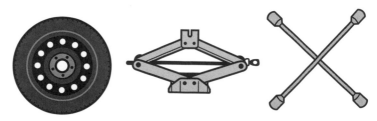

the flat tire by turning counterclockwise once on each nut. You may first have to remove a hubcap covering these nuts by using a flat-head screwdriver to pry it off the wheel, though some lug wrenches feature a flat end for this purpose.

3. *JACK IT UP*

Take your car jack and place it under the part of your car's frame near the flat tire. The exact best position for your car will be found in your owner's manual, but know that you never want the jack to hit the axel or suspension member. The vehicle should have notches on its underside specifically made for a jack, so, again, your manual is your guide when discovering these locations. Once you've positioned the jack where it needs to go, raise it until your vehicle is about six inches higher than when you started.

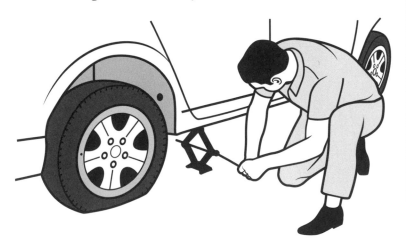

4. *TIRE OFF*

Grab your lug wrench again, this time removing the lug nuts completely. Make sure you place the nuts somewhere you won't lose them, as you'll need them later. Now grab the tire by its treads and pull it off the wheel. When you're completely finished changing the tire and have lowered it back to the ground, you can place the flat in your car to dispose of later.

5. *TIRE ON*

Grab your spare and line it up with the lug bolts on the wheel hub before placing it. Once the bolts and rim are aligned, gently push the spare onto the hub. Take your lug wrench and the lug nuts you carefully placed somewhere and loosely screw on the nuts (about one turn each).

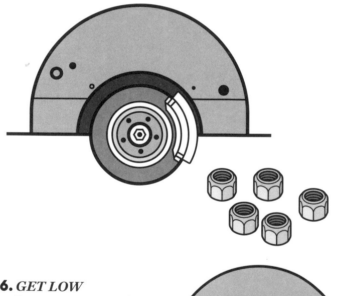

6. *GET LOW*

Return to your jack and carefully lower your car back to the ground. Tighten the lug nuts all the way, put your tools away, and you're ready for the road! Just

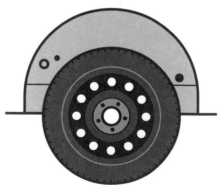

note that if your spare tire is smaller than a normal tire (which is common), you'll want to drive a little slower than usual. You should find a place to change out the spare with a regular tire as soon as you can, as the spare will wear out quicker than a standard one.

HOW TO PREVENT A FLAT TIRE

You may know how to change your tire without pulling out the AAA card, but chances are you would rather be doing something with your time other than switching out a flat. Here are a few simple steps you can take to avoid a flat tire and keep on keeping on.

1. Check the air pressure of each of your tires every month. And by checking the pressure, we mean use an air pressure gauge to make sure the PSI matches what your manual says it should. Just eyeballing the wheels isn't enough.

2. Rotate your tires every 5,000 miles. A vehicle's weight isn't distributed evenly on the wheels, causing the treads on some tires to wear out quicker than others if not rotated. Worn out treads = flat tire, so be on the lookout.

3. Don't overload your vehicle with too much weight. You should be able to find the tire's load measuring index number on the sidewall, which you can take to a mechanic (or look up online) to find the maximum load it can bear.

HOW TO CHANGE YOUR OIL

 MAN'S VEHICLE IS his chariot that carries him from adventure to adventure on the open road. Don't you think you should know how to change your chariot's oil?

1. *GET READY*
Before you start unscrewing valves and mucking around in your engine, gather your supplies first. You'll need:

- *Oil,* about 4 to 6 quarts of the stuff, and make sure it's the type of oil specified in your owner's manual
- *A new oil filter*
- *2 wrenches,* a drain plug socket wrench and an oil filter wrench
- *A large drain pan,* at least 5 to 7 quarts in capacity
- *Rags*
- *A funnel*
- *Safety glasses*
- *Wheel ramps and wheel blocks*

2. *NOW GET THE VEHICLE READY*
Make sure your ride is on steady, level ground and then drive your front wheels up the ramps to elevate the top part. Turn on your parking brake and place wheel blocks behind the rear wheels for added safety. This is an easier way of giving you enough room under your vehicle to work with than using a jack and has the added bonus that you don't have to worry about decapitation. Have your car idle for about 10 minutes before turning it off. Your goal is to work with oil that's not too hot, but isn't cold either, like a greasemonkey Goldilocks.

3. *DRAIN IT*

Pop the hood of your car to access the engine and find the oil filler cap. Turn this cap so it's loose and breaks the vacuum, which makes draining the oil easier. Slide under the front of the car and locate the oil drain plug. Look for a big bolt on the oil pan, which is the large pan-looking object on the underside of the vehicle. Referring to your manual will be a huge help in locating everything. Loosen the drain plug by hand or with a wrench and then place the drain pan you brought with you under the plug where you can see the oil will drain. Once everything is in position, release the drain plug but keep a good grip on it so it isn't washed into the drain pan by the ensuing stream of oil.

4. *NO FILTER*

While the old oil is draining into your pan, pop back topside and find the oil filter in the engine of the vehicle (again, your manual is your friend). Turn it counterclockwise to remove it, and dump any oil inside into your drain pan. Then grab your new oil filter and screw it in where the old one was. Applying a thin layer of new oil to the edge of the filter will help seal it to the gasket to ensure a good fit. Go back under the car and screw the oil plug back into its proper place on the oil pan.

5. *FILL 'ER UP*

Take your funnel and place it in the oil filter under the hood of the vehicle. Pour in the amount of new oil specified in your owner's manual and check afterward with a dipstick to make sure you've filled your vehicle with the correct amount. Replace the cap on the oil filler, close the hood and you're ready for the road—almost.

6. *PROPER DISPOSAL*

You don't want to just chuck the old oil into your backyard. Pour the old oil into a sealable container and drop it off at your local auto shop, which should dispose of it for you at no cost.

HOW TO PROPERLY PAINT A WALL

F YOUR HOME IS your castle, why leave the task that gives it the most personality to a stranger? If you have the time and the gumption to take on the challenge of painting a wall yourself, you'll discover you don't need to be da Vinci to do a good job. Check out the instructions below and get ready to make your mark.

1. *CLEAR AND COVER*
Make sure any furniture in the room you're painting is either moved out of the way or covered by a tarp to prevent stains. Don't forget to put down a drop cloth on the floor beneath your wall. Putting some painter's tape on the wall's trim and on the ceiling along the edges where it meets the wall will also save you time at the end of the day.

2. *CLEAN UP*
Before you apply primer you're going to want to make sure your wall is properly cleaned. Grab a warm, wet cloth and gently wipe down the surface area, then let it dry.

3. *ROLL OUT*
Pour some primer in a paint tray and roll your paint roller in it. Now roll an even coat of it onto the wall, from top to bottom. You should cover any leftover gaps along the trim, ceiling and corners by using a regular paint brush. Just make sure the coat is even so that the paint will be able to stick. Wait about four hours for the

primer to dry (that's enough time to watch *True Grit* and *Rooster Cogburn* and still have time to make a sandwich in between). Alternatively you can buy paint and primer in one, but if your walls are dark and you're using a lighter color, you'll want to prime ahead of time.

4. *STIR THINGS UP*
Once the wall is dry you're going to want to stir your paint so it's even. Take a paint mixer and stir the paint until it has a smooth consistency. This will ensure the finish comes out well.

5. *SECURE THE PERIMETER*
Take your paint brush and dip it into the bucket, making sure to remove any excess paint. Use long, smooth strokes to paint the outer corners of the wall. Do this until the entirety of the wall's perimeter has been outlined.

6. *OUTSIDE IN*
Now it's time to use the roller again. Pour your paint into a clean paint tray (or fresh paint tray liner) and roll the paint roller into the paint, dragging it over the upper, slanted portion of the paint tray to remove excess paint, which helps prevent drips. Begin painting the wall in an "M" pattern to keep the paint even. If you want to apply separate coats, be sure to wait at least two hours so that the previous one dries.

7. *TOUCH UP*
Check the wall and ceiling for any unseemly marks or mistakes before you pack up your supplies. Then carefully remove your painter's tape. It will take about a day or two for the paint to fully dry.

HOW TO SHAVE WITH A STRAIGHT RAZOR

N ODD MUSTACHE or 5 o'clock shadow aside, John Wayne wasn't one to regularly sport facial hair. While there's nothing wrong with growing a beard, those wanting to go clean-shaven like Duke should consider ditching whatever dinky, 10-blade plastic abomination they currently use to scrape their faces and pick up a sharp, straight-edge razor instead. Not only does a straight-edge efficiently cut hair at the skin's surface, avoiding the pulling and tugging that causes irritation and ingrown hairs, it looks damn impressive—even if you're the only one watching.

1. *STROP IN*
Before you start shaving, you'll want to strop and hone your blade so it's ready to slice through your facial hair. Hold the razor with your fingertips, and then lay it flat on a leather strop (which you can purchase online or at any store carrying traditional shaving products). Both the sharp edge of the razor and the back of the razor should be in contact with the strop. Without using too much pressure, pull the razor toward you (with the back of the blade leading, not the cutting edge unless you want to slice up your strop). As you pull, you should angle the blade about 30 degrees to the strop. Once you've pulled the razor the length of the strop, flip the blade and

perform the same motion away from you toward the other end of the strop. Repeat about five times and you should have a new, sharp edge to your blade.

2. GET PREPPED
The first step of a straight razor shave doesn't involve the blade at all, but your face. Either take a hot shower or apply a towel soaked in hot water to your face and neck for a couple of minutes to soften your facial hair and open your pores. If you want, dab a few drops of pre-shave oil in your hands and rub it into your wet face for extra glide. Then take your preferred shaving cream or soap and apply it to your face with either your hands or a brush in a circular motion.

3. GRAB HOLD
Take hold of the razor in a way that gives you complete control over its movement—for many people, that means grasping the razor mostly by the blade (rather than the handle) with the thumb resting just below the edge of the blade and the index, middle and ring fingers resting on the other side of the blade.

4. KNOW ALL THE ANGLES
Tilt the razor so it cuts at roughly a 30-degree angle to your skin—too steep and you'll slice through your skin, too shallow and you won't cut efficiently. Use your free hand to stretch the skin taut and gently make a pass with the razor in the same direction your beard grows (known as "with the grain"). It's absolutely essential to use zero pressure while cutting and rely on the weight of the razor to get the job done.

5. KEEP CUTTING (HAIR, NOT SKIN)
Continue your with-the-grain pass, adjusting the razor when necessary around your lip, jawline and neck to ensure you are shaving in the same direction as hair growth. Don't go over the same area of skin twice, even if stubble is still left. When you're done, wash your face

and assess your shave. Is it as close as you want? Great, we're done here. If not, read on.

6. *AGAINST THE FLOW*
If you want a closer shave, re-apply shaving cream and soap and go for another pass. For many men, another pass with the grain gets them where they want to be. The more swarthy among us may need to take a pass either across the grain or even against the grain. Not everyone's skin can take an against-the-grain pass without irritation, so proceed with caution and don't lose heart if your face doesn't resemble the buttocks of a baby—it's just a sign of your off-the-charts manliness.

7. *KEEPING YOUR EDGE*
After several shaves, you'll find your straight razor tugs and pulls rather than slices, a surefire sign that its edge has dulled. Fortunately, you can solve this problem by honing the razor with a whetstone before stropping. Take the razor and lay it flat against the stone, then run it sharp-edge first down the stone once, flip it, and run it sharp-edge first in the opposite direction. Make sure to keep the razor absolutely flat against the stone, otherwise you can warp the edge. After a couple of passes, strop the razor and you'll be ready to roll.

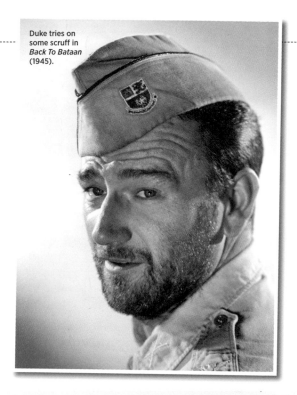

Duke tries on some scruff in *Back To Bataan* (1945).

HOW TO TAKE CARE OF A BEARD

Say you prefer a more rugged appearance over a clean-shaven one. Does that mean you can just let your beard get as weird as it wants to be? Maybe if you're Grizzly Adams. If you aren't, heed the following advice on how to rock that lumberjack look.

1. Wash your facial hair. Some people treat beards like they melt when met with water. Those people also have smelly beards, so wash it with shampoo and add a conditioner as well to ensure facial hair you can be proud of.

2. Trimming your beard is also something you should consider, even if you are trying to grow it out. You can do this the old-school way with scissors, but electric trimmers are relatively inexpensive and make it easy to get rid of wild strays and shape the beard in whatever way you desire.

3. Brush your beard, unless you are trying to go for the look where people think you're carrying around small woodland creatures in there.

HOW TO FIX A LEAKY FAUCET

 HERE ARE A LOT OF reasons you don't want a leaky faucet in your home. Not only does it waste water, the defective plumbing fixture also creates a distracting noise. But the real offense lies in the fact that with every errant drop of water, your abilities as a homeowner are belittled. It's a challenge you shouldn't have to put up with, and thanks to the help of this illustrated guide, you don't have to.

While there are four main types of faucets commonly found in American households, the most likely culprit when it comes to a leak is a compression faucet as it includes parts most easily damaged by ordinary use. Let's walk you through how to put a stop to the drip-drip-drip and restore your deserved peace and quiet.

1. *SHUT IT DOWN*

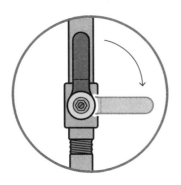

First things first—you need to shut off the water to the faucet in question before you go around digging in its guts. Check under the sink to find the water supply valve. Turn the valve shut (most likely by twisting in a clockwise direction). Once water has been cut off to the faucet, turn on the faucet to make sure any remaining water in the pipes is expelled.

2. *HANDLE IT*

You'll need to remove both handles to figure out which one is responsible for the leak. Pry off any decorative

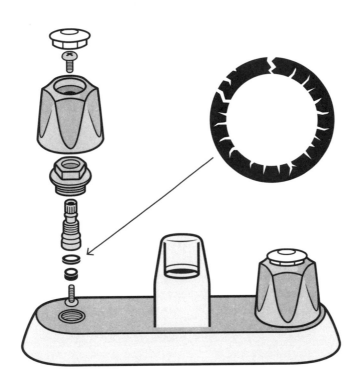

caps on the handle to expose a screw. Take a Phillips-head screwdriver and remove the handles. Now you can take a pair of pliers and remove the nut holding the stem assembly of the handle to the sink. It's this stem assembly that you'll want to focus on in the next steps.

3. *EAGLE EYE*
Hold the stem assembly in your hand and pay attention to the rubber washer at the end (called the O-ring). An O-ring with any sort of damage prevents a proper seal. Replace the O-ring with a new one (you can easily pick this up from a hardware store) and reassemble the stem assembly and the handle.

HOW TO PROPERLY SET THE TABLE

 HIS MAY COME as a surprise, but some folks take issue with sitting down to a nice home-cooked meal and discovering the table looks like a mish-mash of forks, knives and napkins. If you're ever called upon to make sure the table looks ship-shape next Thanksgiving (or whenever you and your family want to put your best face forward), remember the rules below to get the job done right.

1. *SET THE PLACEMATS*
Before you set down any silverware, you need to lay down a placemat for each person attending. Not only does it look put together, it keeps your table clean and helps prevent scratches from the utensils and plates.

2. *PLACE THE PLATES*
You're ready for your plates. Put each plate in the center of each placemat in order to have room for your utensils and napkin to be added on either side. If you're using bread plates and butter knives, it's easiest to add them once you've set all the silverware. Place the plate above your forks with the butter knives on the plate parallel to the side of the table, with the blade on the left-hand side, facing the forks.

3. *LAY THE NAPKINS*
Place one folded napkin on the left of each plate. Fold it in half diagonally, making it look like a triangle. Have the longest side facing the plate with the widest point facing outward.

4. *FORK, KNIFE AND SPOON, IN THAT ORDER*

Each seat gets all three utensils. Place the fork on top of the napkin (if you're adding salad forks, place them to the left of the larger, standard forks), then place the spoon and knife on the right side of the plate. The knife should be on the inside, closer to the plate, and the spoon should be on the right side of the knife, farther from the plate. Make sure the blade of the knife is facing the plate—you know, so you don't have to flip it over once you're ready to dig in.

5. *ADD YOUR GLASSWARE*

Finally, place the glasses above everything on each placemat. Have the glass aligned between the plate and the knife. If you need a spot for wine glasses, place them to the right of each water glass, above the spoons. Now you have everything set up for some fancy chow.

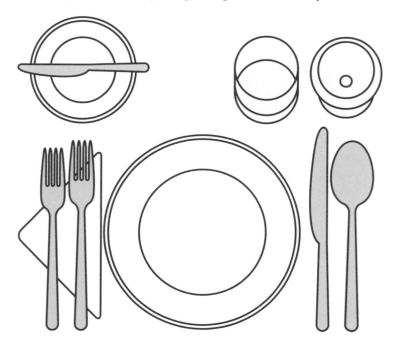

HOW TO CLEAN YOUR BATHROOM IN 10 MINUTES

HE BATHROOM is the one place in your house guests are almost guaranteed to visit, and also the one likely to reveal what a slob you are. Because you've probably neglected giving your bathroom a good, deep clean in favor of more pleasant activities such as doing your taxes or getting a root canal, we've outlined a cheat sheet for making your most holy of holies presentable in just a few minutes. You're welcome.

1. *STRIP IT BARE*
Your first order of business is to remove any towels, toothbrushes, razors, loofahs, etc. from the bathroom in a hurry so nothing is between you and the surfaces that need cleaning. You don't have to be delicate about this—just toss the stuff in another room so you can get to the grimy work of making the bathroom presentable.

2. *SET AND FORGET*
Take your bottle of all-purpose bathroom cleaner and hit up the shower and the inside of the toilet bowl with a hefty amount of sprays. Then take a soft rag, spray it with your cleaner until damp and wipe down the sink, mirror, the outside of the toilet and any other surfaces.

3. *TAKE DOWN THE DIRT*
Now return to the shower, where the dirt and grime has been softened by the cleaner you initially bombarded it with. Take your rag and go to town here, wiping up the dirt and grime until it's presentable. Then head to the

toilet bowl and, using a toilet brush, scrub the inside surface and under the edges, finishing with a flush.

4. *GRACEFUL EXIT*

Before you leave the bathroom, get down on your knees and wipe down the floor with a rag (you could use a mop, but this is the quick version we're going for). That should pick up any excess debriss, dirt and hair from the floor and leave you with a presentable bathroom for your guests to enjoy. Place the towels and other items back in the room and enjoy a job well (or at least quickly) done.

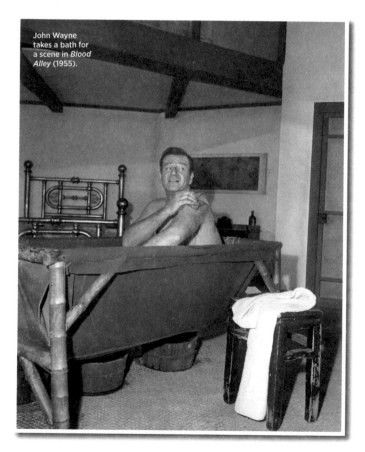

John Wayne takes a bath for a scene in *Blood Alley* (1955).

HOW TO SHINE YOUR SHOES

OTHING ANNOUNCES "I don't pay attention to details" like a pair of scuffed up dress shoes when you're wearing your fancy duds. It's the equivalent of forgetting your hat when going out for a day on the range—it just ain't right. Learn how to avoid this mistake by reading the instructions below.

1. *GATHER YOUR KIT*

The essential tools you'll need to make your shoes mirror-bright include a shoe brush, a soft rag (or an old T-shirt), leather cleaner and conditioner, shoe polish and wax. You can either purchase these items all together as a kit or collect them one by one, but whatever sting you feel at this initial investment will be well worth it when you start receiving compliments left and right on your shiny shoes.

2. *GET THE PAPERS*

Another vital material for shining your own shoes is newspaper, and lots of it. Nothing ruins the satisfaction of a good shoe shine like the realization that you just ruined the furniture and floors of your house. Once you've placed newspaper around your work area, get to work cleaning the dirt and debris clinging to the shoes with your brush. Use some of the leather cleaner if the pair is particularly filthy (no judgements here) and once you're satisfied, remove the shoelaces and get ready to make those puppies pretty.

3. *POLISH*

Take some of the leather conditioner and apply a thin layer to the shoe's surface. Let the conditioner set in for about 10 or even 20 minutes, then take your soft cloth and dab some shoe polish on it. Apply the polish in a circular motion over the entire shoe's surface and remember "less is more." If you feel the shoe needs more polish, you can easily add another layer, but go easy at first, because you'll be surprised how much of a difference a little amount can make. Use a cream polish if you want a softer look, or a wax polish if you really want to turn some heads.

4. *GET BUFF*

Once you've applied the polish, whether cream or wax, buff the shoe with your soft cloth to remove any excess product and enjoy your new, shiny shoes.

HOW TO BUY SHOES THAT FIT

Your shiny new shoes should leave you with a big grin on your face, but that's impossible if you're wearing a grimace of pain from too-tight shoes, or keep tripping over yourself because they're too large. Here are the ins and outs of selecting a perfect fit so you feel like Cinderella every time you go to the store (but in a manly way).

1. Socks matter, in the sense that wearing a pair of thick athletic socks to try on dress shoes won't give you an accurate gauge of whether the pair fits or not. When you're trying on a new pair, make sure the socks you're wearing fit the shoes.

2. Your feet expand throughout the day, so trying on a new pair in the afternoon is preferable to first thing in the morning.

3. When you have the new pair on your feet, check to make sure there's about half an inch from your big toe to the tip of the shoe. Also pay attention to the width. If you feel any pinching, you should size up. Conversely, if you feel you're about to "step out" of the shoe, go a size down.

HOW TO WATERPROOF YOUR DRESS SHOES

 RAINY DAY is no excuse for ruining your best pair of shoes. If you don't want to tie a pair of plastic bags around your feet (and why would you?) then waterproofing your shoes is going to involve applying a layer of protective film that keeps the moisture out without permanently gunking up your gear. Whichever of the below waterproofing materials you choose, apply it to your shoes in the same way you would shoe polish (see page 156). And test a small area of your shoe before dousing the entire thing, just in case of unexpected stains or discoloration.

1. *WATERPROOF COMPOUND*
   There is a vast variety of commercial waterproof compounds out there. The three most common types sold are: specialty waterproofing compounds, spray-on waterproofing compounds and wax-based polishes. Wax-based polishes are your best bet for the ultimate protection. Compared to the spray compound, the wax-base is more durable and allows the leather to breathe.

2. *VASELINE FOR VICTORY*
   Believe it or not, Vaseline isn't just for dry skin or lips. When using it on yourself, it creates a waterproof barrier to the skin and holds in moisture. If you apply this to your leather shoes, it will serve the same

function. And if vaseline is good enough for your lips, isn't it worth trying on your shoes?

3. *MIND YOUR BEESWAX*
Beeswax is also a popular waterproofing method. It provides a strong barrier over the shoe, rather than soaking in. Beeswax won't provide the best shine, and if applied too heavily, it can alter the appearance of your shoe. For easy and light application, make sure you warm up the wax slightly. When it comes to beeswax, less is more.

HOW TO DRY SOAKING WET SHOES

So, you didn't take our advice and waterproof your shoes? Don't worry, we won't take it personally. But do us a favor and follow these tips on how to dry your shoes so they don't end up as an ill-fitting pair that looks and smells like you picked them up from a dump.

1. Use a clean, wet cloth to wipe off any mud or dirt clinging to the shoes.

2. Take out the insole of the shoes (if they are easily removable) and allow them to air dry separately. If you can't separate the insoles from the rest of the shoe, it's nothing to fret over. It may just take a little longer for the shoes to dry.

3. Take some old newspaper and ball it up. Insert the newspaper inside the shoes. Now wrap the outside of the shoes in newspaper and secure with a rubber band.

4. Secure in a dry, warm place and wait for the shoes to dry (it may take a day). Change out the newspaper if it becomes completely sodden until everything is dry.

HOW TO TIE A NECKTIE

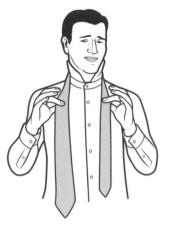

 HERE ARE many ways to wrap a piece of silk or cotton around your neck to look spiffy, but we'll walk you through the most versatile knot that will see you through any situation when wearing a tie is called for—the four-in-hand. This small, unobtrusive knot will dress up any dress shirt while ensuring the attention stays where it belongs—on you and not your tie.

1. *LONG AND SHORT OF IT*

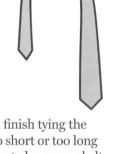

Grab your necktie and face a mirror so you can see what you're doing. Pop your shirt collar and place the tie around the back of your neck along the base of the collar with the front of the tie facing out. The wide end should be on your right side, with the skinny end on your left side. Adjust the tie so the skinny end is slightly above your belly button. After you finish tying the knot, you may discover the tie is either too short or too long for your body (you want the end to hang just above your belt buckle). If necessary, re-tie the tie, placing the skinny end higher on your body if you need a longer tie and closer to your waist if you need to shorten things up.

2. *OVER, UNDER AND UP*

Take the wide end in your hand (the only end you'll actually move) and take it across your body over the skinny end. Then

take the wide end under the skinny end, back across the front
and then up through the loop you've just created (you're gonna
want to look at the beautiful pictures here to help you out).

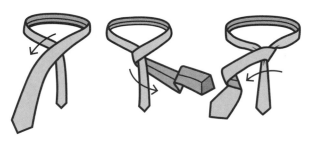

3. *PULL THROUGH
AND PUSH*

There's now a small loop
right in front of you. Take the
wide end of the tie and pull
it through that loop. Most
people would just keep pulling,
tightening the knot and calling
it a day. There's no shame in
that, but if you want to look
like you know what you're

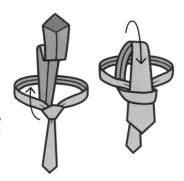

doing, take the index finger of your hand and firmly place
it near the top of the tie where it meets the knot as you pull.
Keep doing this, and you'll create a fashionable dimple in
your finished tie.

4. *KEEP IT TIGHT*

You've tied the knot, but your tie is just sitting in front of your
chest. Grab the skinny part of the tie (which is now concealed
behind the wider part) and pull down to tighten the necktie
to your collar. Make it tight to ensure there's no gap between
your top button and the tie for a more formal look, if that's
what you want. Again, the end of the tie should land just
above your belt buckle, so if you need to start over there's no
shame in it. Flip down your shirt collar and you're done.

HOW TO GRILL A PERFECT STEAK

 RILLING A STEAK isn't just the best way to feed yourself something delicious. It's also an opportunity to demonstrate your culinary credentials to loved ones, friends and anyone else who swings by your backyard BBQs. Become the legend of your neighborhood by following these simple instructions for turning a piece of meat into an edible work of art.

1. *PREPARE THE MEAT*
About a half hour before grilling, take the steak out of the fridge and let it warm up to room temperature. This makes your life easier when attempting to cook it the way you like (Duke ate his rare, but have it your own way). Lightly oil the steak on both sides with your oil of choice and sprinkle both sides with salt, which helps the meat retain moisture to create a juicy dinner.

2. *CAN YOU FEEL THE HEAT?*
Fire up the grill and wait until the flames are a bright, glowing orange. Place your hand 2 inches above the hottest spot on your grill, and if you can hold it there for exactly 2 seconds, you're ready to start! Once your steak hits the grill, you should hear a satisfying sizzle.

3. *CONTROL YOUR FLAMES*
Remember the other side of your grill? The not-so-hot side? If your grill starts to flare up, just slide your steak to that side with your tongs to keep it safe! Many people use a spritz bottle filled with water to control the flame, but

that can kick up ash onto your meat. Ash doesn't taste as good as steak, so that's something you want to avoid.

4. *TOOL TIME*

A thermometer is a crucial and efficient way to ensure you cook the steak to the desired temperature. Reference the below information to find out when you should take your steaks off the grill.

- *Rare* 120 to 130 degrees F
- *Medium Rare* 130 to 135 degrees F
- *Medium* 140 to 150 degrees F
- *Medium Well* 155 to 165 degrees F
- *Well* 170 or higher degrees F

5. *REST UP*

Once your steak is done to your liking, take it off the grill and let it rest for a good 10 minutes. Cover it with some aluminum foil to help preserve the heat of the meat while allowing the juices to spread and settle. Now the only thing left to do is eat the most delicious steak you've ever grilled.

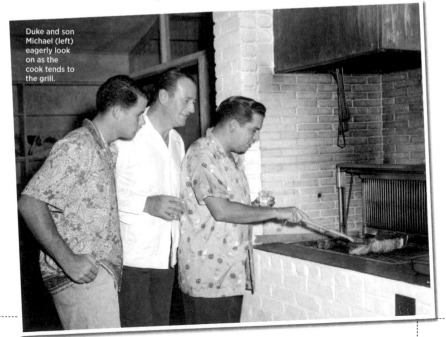

Duke and son Michael (left) eagerly look on as the cook tends to the grill.

HOW TO MAKE YOUR BED MILITARY-STYLE

 URING A COMMENCEMENT SPEECH at The University of Texas at Austin, Adm. William McRaven imparted some advice to the graduating class about what he believed was the most important thing a person can do from day to day. No doubt surprising many in the audience, McRaven's most valuable skill wasn't anything learned in combat, but rather something many of us learn as children: Making a bed. Making one's bed is the perfect task to start the day, imparting an immediate feeling of accomplishment that can lead to a more productive feeling throughout the day. This feeling is even more acute when you take the time to make your bed "by the book," as West Point cadets and recent draftees have done throughout American military history.

1. *PLACE THE FITTED SHEET*
This is the easy part. Just make sure you're not holding it sideways.

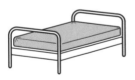

2. *PLACE THE TOP SHEET*
The sheet's wide seam should be at the head of the bed so it's even with the top of the mattress. Tuck in the bottom, leaving the sides free.

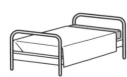

3. *LAY THE BLANKET OVER TOP*

Place the blanket over the top sheet so the sides are uniform in length. (The U.S. insignia, which appears on official military blankets, should face your inspecting officer, who will be looking from the foot of the bed.) Don't pull the blanket all the way up to the top: leave six inches of space between the end of the mattress and the end of the blanket. Tuck the bottom of the blanket in, leaving the sides free as before.

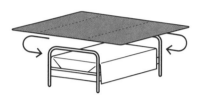

4. *FOLD THE SHEET OVER*

Stretch the blanket to the inner edge of the top sheet's seam. Fold the seam over the blanket. Make an additional fold at the top of the sheet, folding both the blanket and the top sheet to make what should be a familiar-looking border between your blanket and the bare fitted sheet, approximately four inches in width.

5. *CHECK YOUR MEASUREMENTS*

Making one more fold-over of the sheet and blanket should leave you 18 inches between the top of the mattress and the beginning of the top sheet. The sheet/blanket fold should measure eight inches, and there should be four inches between your pillow and the top of the fold.

6. *WRAP IT UP*

Holding the sheet and mattress cover together, fold them completely under the mattress on both sides.

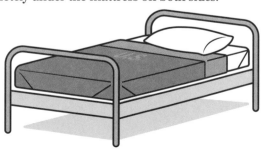

HOW TO PUT OUT A GREASE FIRE

HEN IT COMES to bacon and burgers, grease is good. When it comes to your cholesterol level, grease isn't so great. And when it comes to causing potentially life-threatening fires, grease is awful. A grease fire usually breaks out in the kicthen, one of the most crowded rooms in your house, and the instinct to douse it with water actually makes things worse. Find out how to put out the flames for good by reading the following.

1. *USE AN OUNCE OF PREVENTION*
A grease fire can actually be called an oil fire, as that's what ignites when you crank up the temperature too high. The progression of the fire means the oil goes from boiling to smoking to "Oh my God call 911!" If your pan of stir-fry starts sending out smoke signals, move it off the burner to avoid having to play amateur firefighter later.

2. *SMOTHER IT*
Should you fail to notice the signs of the impending conflagration and find yourself dealing with a full-on grease fire, don't panic (which will be easier said than done). The first thing you should do is turn off the heat. For small grease fires, throwing baking soda into the flames can be enough to squelch the problem. But the surefire method of stopping any grease fire is by starving it of oxygen, which means covering the pan or pot with a metal lid (glass ones can shatter from the heat). Keep it covered until the fire burns itself out.

3. *CHEMICAL WARFARE*

If you don't have anything around the kitchen to smother the fire, or if the inferno is so intense you feel there's no way to safely approach the problem, a good-old fashioned fire extinguisher should take care of the problem. Follow the instructions on the fire extinguisher (hint: it involves pointing and spraying) and your fire will be kaput. You'll have to deal with cleaning up a kitchen covered in chemicals, but that's far better than having to find a hotel for the night.

HOW TO SURVIVE A FIRE

Let's say that grease fire gets out of hand (which it really shouldn't if you follow the preceding instructions, but hey, stuff happens) or your house is on fire for other, non-culinary reasons—you need to escape. If you're reading this book, we can assume you aren't currently in the middle of an inferno, so take the time now to plan your escape route and go over it with your family. Try and follow these tips to make sure you and yours make it to safety.

1. Let everyone else in the house know it is currently on fire. If you're smart, your house is equipped with smoke alarms on every floor that should alert everyone of the situation. If

not, shame on you. Make sure people are apprised of the situation by telling them (or even just yelling "fire!").

2. Quickly but calmly make your way to an exit. Check closed doors with the back of your hand before opening them—if you feel heat at the top or bottom of the door, or at the crack between the door and the frame, find another way out. Consider having an emergency ladder on hand in case your only option is a window.

3. Stay low to the ground, crawling if necessary, to avoid breathing in as much smoke as possible. Most fire-related deaths are from smoke-inhalation, so take this tip seriously.

HOW TO CHANGE A DIAPER

 HE LINE SEPARATING the rugged individualist from the less-than-capable is a willingness to get the job done, no matter how dirty. And it doesn't get any filthier than changing the diaper of a baby who may look sweet and innocent, but somehow possesses the bowels of a much older, smellier human. The next time your little bundle of joy decides to fill 'er up, don't panic: you've got this.

1. *SIMMER DOWN*

To keep the baby safe and comfortable, lay the infant down on a flat surface. This will not only help the baby be comfortable, but it will also make sure the job is clean and easy. Have a new, clean diaper and some baby wipes within reach for easy access. Make sure your diaper is already open so you don't waste time opening it while cleaning the baby. You should also have some baby powder or aloe lotion if you see the baby has a diaper rash. Having all these things handy will make changing his or her diaper very easy and quick.

2. *THE DIRTY WORK*

It's time to do some dirty work. You're finally situated with everything you need. Undo the baby's clothes to fully show the diaper. Undo the sticky straps on the front of the diaper to open it up. Don't be intimidated by the mess, everything will be OK—you have wipes. Lift up the baby's legs and take a wipe or two (or 10) to clean the backside. Once the backside is clean, keep the legs up, slide the dirty diaper out from under the baby's bottom and put the new one in its place. Then clean the front side of the baby with a fresh wipe.

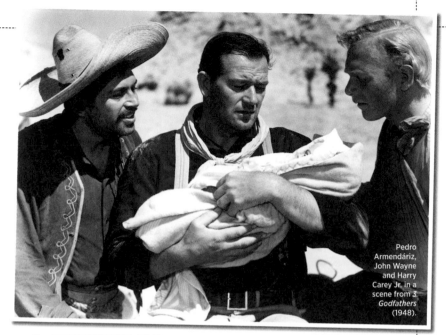

Pedro Armendáriz, John Wayne and Harry Carey Jr. in a scene from *3 Godfathers* (1948).

3. *FINISH THE JOB*

Now that your baby is all clean, check for any sign of rash. If your baby's skin looks a bit irritated because of the diaper, get some baby powder or aloe lotion and apply it to the affected area before strapping on the new diaper. Once that's done, pull the front part of the diaper up between the baby's legs and hold it gently against the belly. Then pull the straps on the back half of the diaper up one at a time and stick them securely to the front of the diaper to hold the whole contraption in place—not too tight, but firmly enough to ensure nothing leaks out between now and the next changing. Now dress the baby back up and let him or her go about the normal business of being a baby.

4. *CLEAN UP TIME*

To dispose of the dirty diaper, roll it upward and use the sticky straps to secure it shut. Get a plastic bag you'd get from the grocery store and put the diaper in the bag. Tie it up and throw it in the trash. You're a diaper changing pro.

HOW TO IRON A DRESS SHIRT

EING AN INDEPENDENT, self-sufficient individual means you focus on what's truly important in life, unconcerned with the frivolities and distractions bogging down the brains of most people. Personal appearance, however, should be filed under the former and not the latter. That doesn't mean you have to get dandied up all the time, but you should always be able to present a clean, competent front to the world when called for. Learning how to properly iron a dress shirt goes a long way toward letting others know you mean business, even when you're wearing it for pleasure.

1. *GET ON BOARD*

You need a sturdy and flat place to iron if you're going to do it right. Set up your ironing board in a comfortable spot before you begin. If you plan on ironing multiple shirts, consider setting yourself up in front of the television.

2. *GEAR UP YOUR IRON*

Fill your iron with distilled or bottled water. Tap water contains minerals that can build up and clog the iron over time (if your iron ever spits a large amount of water, it's clogged!). Set your iron to the correct setting, depending on your shirt's condition as well as the care instructions on its tag. If it's very wrinkled, put your iron at the highest setting and set the steam for "high" as that also helps get rid of stubborn wrinkles (assuming your shirt's care instructions don't forbid both). If your shirt is slightly wrinkled, put it on a cooler setting below its max. Set the iron on its base so the metal part is facing outward as it heats up.

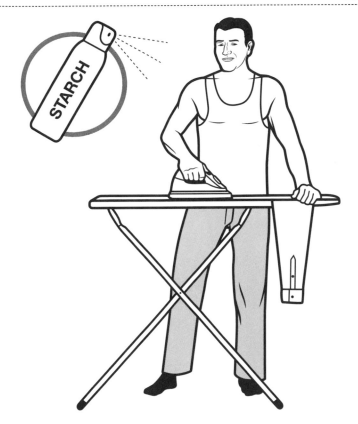

3. *HANGING OUT*

As your iron heats up, prepare a space to hang up your ironed shirt(s) once you're finished. Do not fold them, or else you will have creases. You don't want to do all that work for nothing!

4. *CONSIDER ADDING STARCH*

This step is optional, but it's useful if you're going for a more formal, dressed-up look. You can buy it in aerosol form, but an easy way to make it at home is to dissolve one tablespoon of cornstarch in two cups of water and add your mixture to a spray bottle. Spray this on your shirt(s) before you start ironing to get a crisp, smooth finish. Make sure you don't overdo it, or else you'll be left with a shirt covered in flakes!

5. *HOT UNDER THE COLLAR*

Now that you have all your tools set up, you can start getting rid of those wrinkles. If you're seeking a super crisp finish, iron your shirt inside out and then turn it back to iron the outside by using the following steps. You will want to iron the collar first. Make sure it is laying flat on the board, and iron from its points to the back of the neck. Don't go too fast or press too hard because you could burn your shirt.

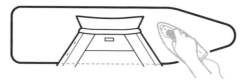

6. *ON THE CUFF*

Lay your cuffs flat and unbuttoned on your board, and start ironing from the inside out. Move all the wrinkles out to the edges. Never iron over the buttons! Make sure you carefully iron around them using the iron's pointed tip as a guide, or else the iron will leave marks.

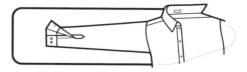

7. *FRONT AND CENTER*

It's time to iron the front of your shirt. Have your shirt unbuttoned, and start ironing on the side with the buttons. Maneuver around them by using the tip of your iron. Then, go back up and iron down the shirt slowly. Repeat this on the other side. If you have a pocket, it can be a bit tricky. Use the tip of your iron for precision and avoid ironing over the seams. Also, if your shirt is printed, iron in the direction of the print or pattern. For example, if if has vertical stripes, iron the shirt vertically.

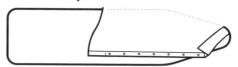

8. *BACK IT UP*

Flip your shirt over, and start ironing the back. Lay your unbuttoned shirt flat, and line up the back of one shoulder to the narrow end of the ironing board, making sure the edge of the board is along the side of your shirt. You should have one half of the back flat on the board for you to iron. After you're done with that one side, you can slide the other side of the shirt to be ironed.

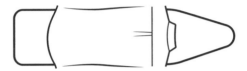

9. *SMOOTH SLEEVES*

Finally, iron your sleeves—one at a time. The key to this step is to make sure your sleeve is fully flat and smooth before you start ironing. When it's finally flat, start ironing from where the sleeve is sewn to the shirt, and follow the seam downward toward the cuff. Turn it over to iron the other side identically as before, and do the same thing to the other sleeve.

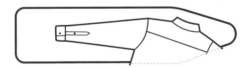

10. *INSPECTION*

Now that you're done ironing, inspect your shirt to make sure you smoothed out all the creases. If you missed a spot, go back and iron. Once it's fully smooth, hang it up on a hanger and button it all the way up. Your shirt is now perfectly ironed and ready to be worn!

HOW TO COOK THE ONLY THREE MEALS YOU NEED

K, YOU PROBABLY will want to expand your diet beyond what's listed below. But these quick and easy recipes can also be customized in numerous ways, making them great go-tos when you need to rustle up some grub.

1. *OMELET*

Beat together 2 eggs, 2 tablespoons of water and a dash of salt and pepper in a mixing bowl. Melt 1 teaspoon of butter in a skillet over medium-high heat until it's hot. Pour in your egg mixture. After 30 seconds or so, when the bottom of the eggs have set, place your choice of filling on one side of the omelet. Shredded cheddar, ham, cooked bacon, spinach, mushrooms and peppers are all good choices—just be mindful not to add more than you can fit. Fold the omelet over the fillings with your spatula and cook for a minute or so more. Flip the omelet, let cook for one more minute, then slide it onto your plate to eat.

2. *AGLIO E OLIO*

This dish sounds fancy, but it's dead simple to make. "Aglio e olio" (pronounced ahl-ee-oh ay oh-lee-oh) is Italian for garlic and oil, and that's all you'll need to make this simple pasta dish.

First, get a pot of salted water boiling. While you're waiting for that to heat up, start mincing your garlic—

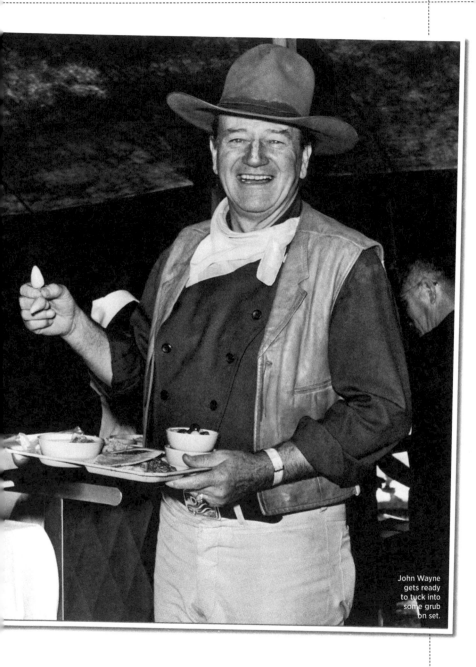

John Wayne gets ready to tuck into some grub on set.

aim for one clove per person, or more if you're a real garlic lover. (We don't recommend making this before a date.) Once the water is boiling, add your pasta. The classic choice is spaghetti, but any noodle you have on hand will do. Cook according to the package directions.

While the pasta is cooking, heat another pan over medium-low and add a few healthy glugs of olive oil. Add your minced garlic and watch it carefully—you're going for a toasty brown. If you like things spicy, add a few pinches of red pepper flakes. Once the garlic is browned, turn off the heat. Using a slotted spoon or tongs, add the cooked pasta directly to the pan with the warm garlic oil and toss it all together, adding more oil if things are looking a little dry. Congratulations, you've just made classic aglio e olio.

Note: To make this more of a "complete" meal, sauté some greens and shrimp or diced chicken before browning your garlic. Continue as directed, then add your extras to the finished product.

3. *COWBOY CHILI*

A classic one-pot, stick-to-your-ribs kind of meal, chili is something every man should know how to make. Start by roughly chopping an onion, a bell pepper and a clove or two of garlic. Heat a large pan over medium, drizzle in some olive oil and add your vegetables. Once they're soft, push them to the side of the pan and add a pound of ground beef. Brown the beef, breaking it up as it cooks. Once your beef is browned, add a can of diced tomatoes (juice and all), a drained can of corn and a drained can or two of black beans or kidney beans. Season with a tablespoon or so of chili powder, a teaspoon of cumin if you have it, and salt and pepper to taste. You can also add a little cayenne, diced habanero or red pepper flakes if you like your chili to have a little heat. Now you have a classic chili that can be scooped up with tortilla chips, piled on a hot dog, covered with cheese and sour cream or enjoyed any other way you like—eat up, pilgrim.

HOW TO CLEAN UP AFTER COOKING

There are few things in life as satisfying as tucking into a meal you've cooked yourself, but there are also few sights as disheartening as a pile of unwashed pots and pans waiting for you after the meal. Follow these tips to cut down on the time you have to spend in the kitchen cleaning, so you can focus more time and energy on what you would rather be doing (which unless you have weird hobbies, is probably almost anything else).

1. Soak your dishes as you go, if possible. It may be impractical to fill the sink with warm, soapy water if you need it during meal prep, but if not, dropping whatever dirty equipment in there to soak as soon as you're finished with it helps make cleaning later a whole lot easier. At the very least, soak everything in suds after you're done cooking and before you start eating.

2. Wipe stains and spills as you go, instead of putting them off for some marathon cleaning session at the end of the night.

3. Cut down on the number of utensils and containers you use. That doesn't mean using the same cutting board for raw meat and veggies, but consolidate when you can.

HOW TO SEW ON A BUTTON

 URE, YOU MIGHT think sewing a button is an uninteresting skill, but if a button pops off your shirt or pants while you're out and about, it's a technique you'll wish you'd mastered. Here are a few simple steps to sew a button up quick and easy.

1. *GATHER AND CUT*
First off, get some supplies. You're going to need a sewing needle, thread, a button and a pair of scissors or a pocket knife. Unspool about a forearm's length of thread, then cut it off cleanly.

2. *THREAD THE NEEDLE*
Feed the thread through the needle's eye. Tie a small knot so the needle is attached to the thread. Tie another knot at the opposite end of the thread.

3. *BUTTON UP*
Now place the button on top of the area you need to sew it onto. Take your needle and stab it through the underside of the cloth, pushing it through one of the button's holes. Pull the thread all the way through, stopping when the knotted end is flush against the cloth.

4. *KEEP ON GOING*
Take your needle and insert it through the hole diagonal to the one you just pulled it through. Always remember to pull the entire needle and thread through the hole so that the thread is pulled tight. Repeat this process for the two remaining holes so the thread is looped tightly in the button's interior. If your thread is thin, sew it through each hole multiple times to make sure it's secure.

5. *PUSH IT*

After you've made your final pass through and the needle is on the interior of the fabric, carefully slide it between the intersection of sewn thread and the fabric. Pull tight and repeat, this time leaving a little slack. Insert the needle through the loop you've created and pull tight to tie off a knot. Cut the thread above the knot. Problem solved.

HOW TO GET RID OF A COFFEE STAIN ON YOUR SHIRT

Popping a button isn't the only way your wardrobe can suddenly betray you. Nothing can turn you from suave to slob quicker than a blot of coffee staining your crisp white shirt. Here are some general first-response tips to help you get rid of that unsightly stain and back to looking your best.

1. Blot the stain as quickly as possible with a paper towel or a clean cloth. You want to remove any excess liquid still hanging around the cloth before moving on to treat the stain itself.

2. Remove the shirt (where and when it is appropriate, of course) and run the stain under cold water. Make sure you are washing the back of the stain (the side that isn't facing everyone when you wear the shirt), pausing every two to three minutes to blot the stain until it is gone.

3. For some extra oomph, dab some dish-washing soap on the stain while you are running it under cold water. If that doesn't do the trick, you might have to live with the stain. Hey, it happens to everyone.

HOW TO PATCH A ROOF

MAN'S HOUSE IS his castle, and no king wants to live in a broken-down palace with a leaky roof. How the rugged individualist goes about repairing small holes or damage largely depends on the type of roof over his head, but we're focusing on shingle roofs. It's one of the most popular types of roofing in the U.S. of A., and repairing a hole in rolled roofing is often as simple as troweling in roof cement over the hole, nailing down that patch and covering those nails with more roofing cement. But don't worry—we'll break down how to take care of a shingled roof so it's just as easy.

1. *PREPARE YOURSELF*
Because the last thing you want to discover when on the roof of your house is that you forgot a vital tool or piece of equipment, take the time to assess what you need to repair the hole. For a shingled roof, that includes:

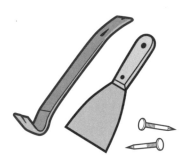

- *A pry bar*
- *A tab of replacement shingles*
- *A putty knife or similar cutting tool*
- *7/8" roofing nails* (the number depends on the amount of shingles you need to replace, with the rule of thumb being around two per shingle)
- *A hammer*
- *Roofing cement*

Safely climb onto your roof, and make your way over to the damaged area of the roof.

2. *OUT WITH THE OLD*

Before you can patch the leaky roof, you first need to get rid of the damaged shingles. Lift up the broken shingle with your hands and use your pry bar to remove the nails holding it to the roof. You may first need to use your knife to cut away any roofing cement helping to keep the shingle in place. Set the damaged shingle (or shingles) aside to take down with you for safe disposal.

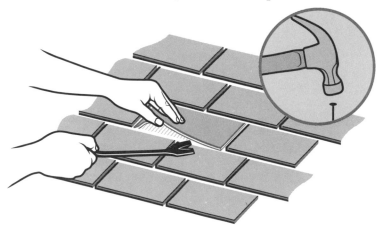

3. *CUT IT OUT*

Take your replacement shingle material, and use your knife to cut new shingles to fit. Slide the new shingles into the spots where the old, damaged ones used to be. Hammer a nail into the top two corners of the shingle to hold it in place, then cover the nails with roofing cement.

HOW TO GET YOUR KIDS TO GO TO BED

 OUR JOB AS A PARENT often consists of getting your children to do things that are in their best interest, particularly when they don't want to do them. When it comes to bedtime, most children hold a strong opinion (hint: it's usually not favorable). Here's how to get them into bed without resorting to tossing them over your shoulder like a sack of potatoes.

1. *TAKE YOUR TIME*

Kids respond very well to having a set routine. It gives their lives order and helps them get into an easily memorizable pattern. Setting up a bedtime that never changes will get the kids into the mindset that there's a specific time for sleep. Kids need more than nine hours of sleep every night so setting this up at a good and early time, like 7 or 9 p.m., will ensure they aren't disrespectful by the morning. Do not compromise on this deadline—set it and stick to it because any breaks could throw off your child's entire sleeping schedule.

2. *DON'T NEGOTIATE*

Kids will always try to weasel out of sleep. They'll say they want you to read the story one more time, or that they need to eat something else, or any number of excuses. Even the time honored, "just stay with me until I fall asleep," is a ploy to keep themselves awake longer. Try and be aware of these demands and don't give in to them. You'll only be doing yourself a disservice in the long run if you humor them.

3. *ACTIVITIES!*

The human mind responds very well to repetition. Don't be afraid to set up a few very specific rituals that you perform every night because this will prepare the mind for sleep. Reading to them or any other soothing activity not only lets them know it's bedtime, but can also be something you both look forward to.

4. *LAY DOWN THE LAW*

When it comes down to it, you are the parent and your word is law. If your child refuses to go to bed, tell them the consequences and then follow through with them. You have the authority to reprimand them and take away privileges, and need to show them you'll use it if necessary. After all, as Duke said in *Rio Grande* (1950), a man's word is his honor.

HOW TO STOP A TANTRUM

Becoming a parent means taking on a whole new heap of worries and fears about your child, most of them fortunately never coming to pass. One that almost certainly will is your little tyke having a nuclear meltdown in public that sends onlookers either scurrying for cover or standing transfixed in horror at what they're witnessing. Here are some tips to diffuse the situation fast.

1. Stay calm. You need to be a pillar of strength and reassurance for your kid who is currently losing it. Don't be that parent who gets in a screaming match with a child. Just don't.

2. If possible, figure out what's bothering your bundle of rage and help him or her solve the problem. Is the child having trouble finding his or her favorite toy? Calmly state that you will help find it.

3. That said, don't give in to demands if the kid is throwing a tantrum because he or she doesn't want to follow the rules. Remain calm but firm in your convictions and, if possible, remove your child from the source of the frustration.

HOW TO BUILD A HOUSEHOLD BUDGET

 ONEY ISN'T EVERYTHING, but it certainly helps. We might not all be blessed with millions, but everyone can (and should) make a basic budget for the household to control wayward expenses and make sure you aren't on a first-name basis with your bill collectors. Read the below tips on what you need to do to stay in the black by keeping track of your green.

1. *GET THAT PAPER*

Before you can start allocating how much money you can spend on a new car or premium cable or whatever else your heart desires, you first need a handle on how much money is coming into your household. That means gathering pay stubs, bank statements and any other records that keep track of income earned. Calculate your total take home pay for a month, which is the sum of any income after taxes, insurance payments and other withholdings. It also means keeping track of how much money leaves your household, from regularly scheduled payments to what you spend on average for food, vacations, etc. Your budget should be your game plan for at least a month, but probably not as long as a year in order to strike a balance between long-term planning and keeping an eye on the more immediate expenses such as monthly bills.

2. *SORT IT OUT*

Now that you have a total number for the money coming in vs. the money going out, break down the outgoing dollars into categories such as mortgage, utilities, groceries, etc. You don't have to go too crazy here—unless you're the Cookie Monster, knowing how much you spend specifically on Oreos every month isn't that helpful. You want to group similar expenses together to see where you are spending most of your money to determine where you can cut back, if necessary.

3. *TIGHTEN THE BELT*

Unlike the government, you can't print your own money (legally), so you need to make sure you have more money coming than leaving the household. Certain expenses are fixed and more difficult to change (such as your rent or mortgage) but others provide a soft target for cost-cutting (e.g., your weekly trip to the Sizzler). Determine what luxuries you can give up before putting a "For Sale" sign in your front yard and remember that as painful as it may be to give up some creature comforts, nothing feels better than not worrying about mounting debt.

HOW TO BREAK BAD SPENDING HABITS

Out-of-control shopping and spending habits can afflict anyone, so don't think that just because you're not coming home from the mall with 20 pairs of shoes that you don't have a problem. If your household budget shows you need to be reaching for the wallet less, there's one trick you can use to put you on the path toward a more frugal lifestyle. Cash is king, although his realm is rapidly shrinking in the age of credit cards, debit cards and online payments. Still, physically handling the money you are about to fork over often makes you reconsider whether you really need that new cowboy hat or set of spurs, allowing you to potentially save for more important purchases like new tires, a replacement water heater or John Wayne books.

HOW TO HAMMER A NAIL

 LENTY OF PEOPLE don't know how to accomplish this simple demonstration of self-sufficiency. Don't be one of them. Read on, and next time you're called upon to do a little carpentry, swing away with confidence.

1. *GET A GRIP*
   Don't hold the hammer like you're ashamed to be here. Grasp the hammer firmly, closer to the head for when you need more control and closer to the end of the handle when you need a dose of power.

2. *EASY DOES IT*
   Hold the nail between your forefinger and thumb (of your non-dominant hand) and place it in the spot you want to drive the nail into. But don't go to town quite yet. Instead, lightly tap the nail until it sticks in the surface without needing to be held.

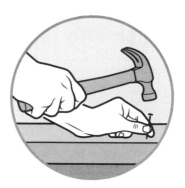

3. *GO WITH THE FLOW*
   Now comes the fun part. Swing the hammer from your elbow to generate more force, but remember you still need to maintain enough control so you are hitting

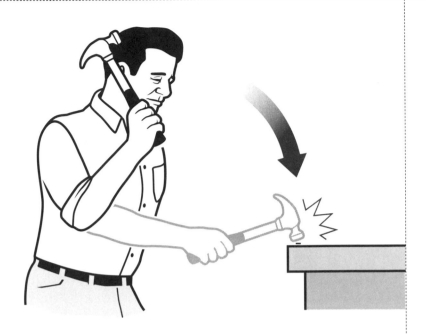

the nail straight on the head (rather than delivering glancing blows that will bend the nail). Tip: Remember you can let the weight and momentum of the hammer do a lot of the work for you, so don't overdo it. You know you're as strong as an ox—no need to prove it on a wimpy piece of metal. You'll know you're finished when the nail is flush with the surface of the wood.

HOW TO PICK A REMODELING CONTRACTOR

 GOOD CONTRACTOR can turn a miserable mess of a home into a magnificent mansion, but a shoddy one can leave you with nothing but a hovel and a pile of bills. Read the tips below to help make the right choice when it comes time to spruce up your digs.

1. *ASK AROUND*
See if any of your friends or family have had good outcomes with past contractors. You can also look into the National Association of the Remodeling Industry. They can show you a list of contractors in the area. Any type of word-of-mouth is a great way to find an amazing and qualified contractor. Ask around at your church, on trusted community message boards or independent home service review sites like Angie's List.

2. *INVESTIGATE*
With some recommendations in hand, investigate and research your candidates. Look on their websites and read reviews from other people who worked with them. See if they have any association with the National Kitchen & Bath Association, the National Association of the Remodeling Industry or the National Association of Homebuilders.

3. *INTERVIEWS*
Set up some interviews for the contractors you favor. Start out with phone interviews. Ask them questions like: Do they work on projects of your size? Are they willing to provide financial references? Are they able to give you a list of previous clients and projects? Will they be

working on other projects? And if so, how many? How long have they been working as a contractor? After you have narrowed it down to about three or four possible candidates, interview them face to face. Make sure you both communicate and work well together.

4. *REACH OUT*
Reach out to former clients, and ask how they worked with the contractor. Also, ask to see the finished product of what they worked on. You can even visit a current job site they are working on to see how they personally work.

5. *GET BIDS AND MAKE A PAYMENT SCHEDULE*
Ask the final contractors to break down the cost of it all. This includes materials, profit margins and labor. Usually, materials make up 40 percent of the total cost. The remaining amount covers the rest, such as overhead and the profit the contractor makes, which is usually 15-20 percent. Once it's all in order, create a payment schedule. It's standard to pay 10 percent up front, followed by a series of equal payments to cover the cost of the job once it's underway. If a potential contractor asks for half or more upfront, it could be a sign that he or she is in financial trouble, which might color your decision on whether or not you let them work on your home.

6. *PUT IT IN WRITING*
Now that you have found your contractor and have agreed on expenses, put it all in writing. Draw up a contract outlining everything you have discussed. It should consist of: a bid price and payment schedule, specifics about the work site plan, a detailed schedule of primary construction tasks, a change-order clause, a written procedure for close-out, and an express limited warranty clause about dispute resolution and a waiver of lien. This waiver will prevent subcontractors and suppliers from putting a lien on a house should the contractor not pay for the materials they use. Once your paperwork is all situated, you're ready for your project to get underway. Shake hands and get to work.

HOW TO COOK AN EGG

IN *McLINTOCK!* **(1963), DUKE** growled, "Don't say it's a fine morning or I'll shoot ya." But would that character still be so grumpy if he had a plate of tasty eggs waiting for him first thing in the a.m.? We doubt it. Make every morning a great one (at least as far as breakfast is concerned) with this how-to guide for cooking eggs.

1. *SCRAMBLED EGGS*
There are a few tricks to get the perfect scrambled eggs, and most of them revolve around the heat. You need to whisk the eggs thoroughly before you cook them. This helps incorporate air into the eggs to make them fluffy. Cook your eggs as you normally would, but turn off the heat before your eggs are fully cooked. This prevents overcooking. No one wants crunchy eggs. For taste, mix in some milk and butter while whisking, and season it up with salt and pepper, to taste.

2. *SUNNY SIDE UP*
The term "Sunny Side Up" comes from the egg's appearance itself. The bright yellow yolk faces up, while the egg white is perfectly fried. Crack open your egg into your pan, and let it fry facing up. Make sure to keep the pan covered until the whites are completely set. This allows the yolk to be nice and runny. You can even dip your toast in the yolk for extra flavor.

3. *OVER EASY*
Remember how it was crucial to not flip your sunny side up egg? Well, when it comes to eggs over easy, that's what you have to do! Cook your egg as if it were

sunny side up, but once the bottom of the whites are set, flip it over. This will cook the top, but it'll keep the center of the yolk runny.

4. *POACHED EGGS*

Poached eggs are notoriously difficult to get just right, but follow these instructions and you'll be a pro. First, fill a pot two-thirds of the way with cold water. Add a teaspoon of vinegar and ½ teaspoon of salt. Bring the water to a gentle simmer. Crack the egg into a small bowl. Reduce the water's heat to low and gently pour the egg in the water. Let it cook for 6 minutes, using a silicone spatula to keep the egg from settling on the bottom of the pot. Remove with a slotted spoon and gently place on a paper towel. Blot off excess water and serve.

5. *HARD BOILED*

Though the name may suggest otherwise, it's actually very easy to cook a hard boiled egg. Just fill a pot with enough water to cover the eggs. Bring the water to a boil and carefully drop the eggs in so that the water doesn't splash and the eggs don't crack on the bottom of the pot. You should leave them in for 10-12 minutes. Then, place the eggs immediately in ice water. This step will make it easier to peel off the shells. Take them out of the cold water and gently tap an egg on the counter until the shell is cracked all over. Roll the egg between your hands to loosen the shell, and start peeling!

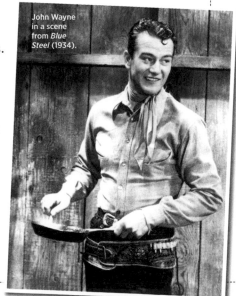

John Wayne in a scene from *Blue Steel* (1934).

HOW TO TREAT A BLACK EYE

 ANY ROADS LEAD to the black eye—a spectacular failure to catch a baseball, a bad run-in with a wall or an unwise comment directed at someone much bigger than you (still—you should see the other guy). However you got your shiner, it needs to be treated, which is why you should use your one good peeper to read the following advice.

1. *CHILL OUT*

The black eye is caused by broken blood vessels under the skin surrounding the eye. Applying a cold compress to the skin will cause those blood vessels to constrict, stopping the bleeding. Your best bet is to take some ice cubes and wrap them in a washcloth, but a bag of frozen veggies or a hunk of cold meat will do. Remember, it's the skin you need cooled off, not the eye itself, so don't bother pressing the compress directly against your eyeball. Hold it to your skin for about 10 minutes once every hour until the swelling goes down.

2. *KEEP AN EYE OUT*

Most black eyes won't necessitate a trip to the doctor's office, but if you spot any of the following warning signs, swallow your pride and seek out some professional medical care: spots of blood in the white part of the eye, severe pain, blurry or double vision. Any of these symptoms could indicate a fracture of the bones surrounding the eye or another serious internal injury.

3. *THAT WARM, FUZZY FEELING*

After about two days, your black eye may look more like a rainbow-colored eye as the bruises change color. You can now start applying a warm compress (which is as easy as taking a washcloth and soaking it in warm-to-hot water) to the skin for 10 minutes every hour to get the blood flowing and jump-start the healing process.

HOW TO STOP A BLOODY NOSE

Again, we're not here to judge why blood is gushing out of your nose—but we can give you some pointers on how to efficiently staunch the flow so you can get back to business.

1. Sit down and lean forward to avoid having blood flow into the back of your throat and into your stomach. Swallowing blood isn't dangerous, but it can often lead to an upset stomach since you aren't a vampire (right?).

2. Pinch your nostrils closed with your thumb and forefinger and keep constant pressure for 10 minutes. After 10 minutes, release your nostrils and see if the bleeding has stopped. If you're still losing blood, pinch for another 10 minutes and see if you have better luck. (And if it doesn't stop after another 10 minutes, seek medical attention immediately.)

3. Take an ice pack or a cold compress and hold it against the bridge of your nose to help stop the bleeding. Do not stuff tissue, gauze or anything else up your nostrils. This actually damages the already-wounded lining of the nose, which can worsen the bleeding.

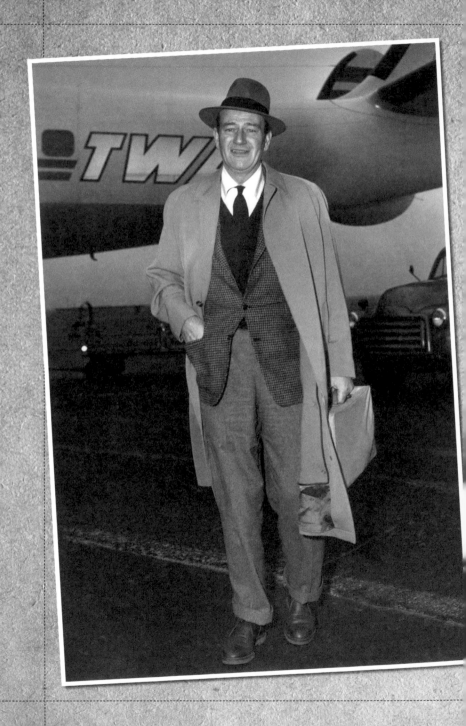

WHEREVER YOU GO

PUT YOUR BEST
FOOT FORWARD, NO
MATTER WHERE LIFE
TAKES YOU

HOW TO SHOOT A RIFLE STRAIGHT

HEN YOU'RE OUT on a hunting trip, you don't want to be the guy who comes back empty-handed while the rest of your buddies are dragging back bucks big enough for them to feast on venison year round. Read the following advice on how to make sure your aim is true. And happy hunting.

1. *EYE TEST*
The first thing you need to figure out is which of your eyes is dominant. Take your hands and make a small triangle (about ½ to ¾ inch per side), overlapping your thumbs to create the base and then laying your left fingers over your right so the first knuckle on each hand's index finger are touching. Look through this triangle at a small object (such as a doorknob) using both eyes. Now shut your right eye. Can you still see the object? Then your left eye is dominant. If you can only see the object with your right eye, then that's the dominant one. In any case, the hand you actually fire the rifle with should be on the same side as your dominant eye.

2. *GET COMFORTABLE*
Finding the right position to keep a steady aim largely depends on what feels right to you. One popular pose is lying prone on your stomach so you can use the ground to help steady your arms. If you don't want to get up-close and personal with the forest floor, you can sit or kneel, using your knee as a support.

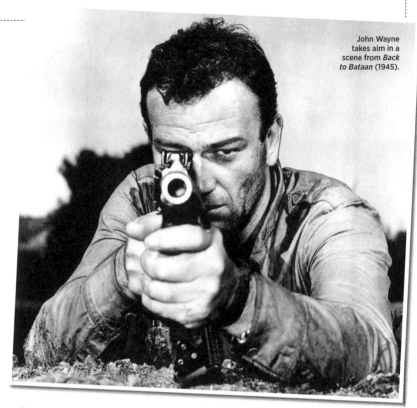

John Wayne takes aim in a scene from *Back to Bataan* (1945).

3. *BUTT TO SHOULDER*

Take the end (called the butt) of the rifle and place it in the hollow between your shoulder on your firing side and your chest. It's important the butt firmly rests on the muscle part of the shoulder—not the armpit and not the collarbone. Otherwise, the recoil of the rifle is going to cause a painful experience.

4. *SHAKE HANDS*

Using your firing hand, grasp the rifle near the trigger stock with a firm grip (as if you were shaking someone's hand), but don't curl your index finger around the trigger itself—you want to keep it nice and straight until the moment you are ready to shoot. Your non-firing hand should be grabbing the rifle farther down the weapon, just short of full extension of your arm, helping to steady the weapon without supporting its weight.

5. *CHEEK TO BUTT*
Naturally bend your neck so the cheek on your firing side rests against the butt of the rifle. This also positions your dominant eye down the barrel (or scope) of the weapon, allowing you to get the target in your literal sights.

6. *PULL THE TRIGGER*
When you're ready to take your shot, remember to squeeze the trigger in a smooth, consistent motion. Don't raise your head too soon and keep your eye on the target during the shot to help ensure you don't make a last-minute move that causes your shot to go astray. With practice, your ability to hit a target will skyrocket.

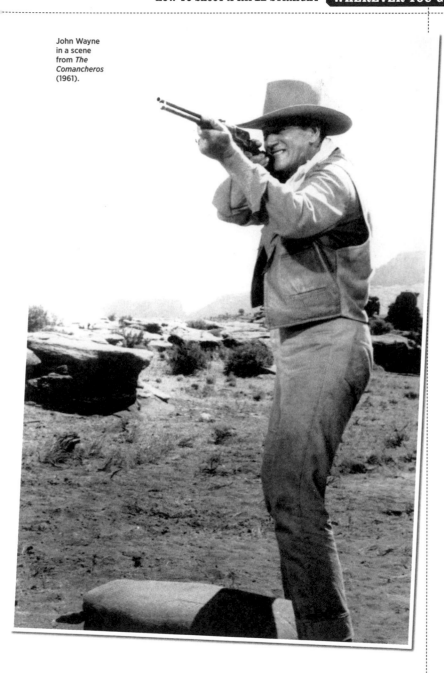

John Wayne
in a scene
from *The
Comancheros*
(1961).

HOW TO THROW A PROPER PUNCH

 S JOHN WAYNE SAID, "I define manhood simply: Men should be tough, fair and courageous, never petty, never looking for a fight, but never backing down from one either." In other words, sometimes despite your best efforts, the only way to solve your problem is with a punch. Better make sure you know how to throw one, pilgrim.

1. *STAND READY*

Unless you've managed to get yourself in a ruckus with a 19th-century dandy, you probably don't have too much time to worry about old-fashioned "fisticuffs" posturing, but that doesn't mean you should ignore it completely. Curl your hands into fists (more on that in a minute) and bring them up to either side of your head to help cover your face from incoming blows. Lower your chin to provide your mug additional protection. Place the foot opposite of your dominant hand (the one you should be punching with) slightly in front of the other one, and bend your knees a little to get in a stance that's both balanced and sets you up for throwing a powerful blow.

2. *FISTS OF FURY*

Don't place your thumb inside your fingers or on the side unless you're trying to leave the fight with a broken hand. You want to strike your opponent with the area of your fist between

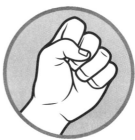

the second and third knuckles of your index and middle fingers (don't worry, follow these instructions and it will come naturally). Your thumbs should hug your first two fingers as illustrated.

3. *STRAIGHT TO THE POINT*

You should focus on delivering short, straight punches packing in as much pain as possible. Keep your elbow tucked in and extend from your shoulder, naturally turning your arm so you'll make contact with the knuckles we mentioned in the step above. At the same time, you should pivot into the punch with your lower body to get the most out of it. Follow-through by punching "through" your target (don't stop extending as soon as you make contact). Don't waste time hitting his jaw or cheek—go for the soft, vulnerable spots such as his nose. Often, a good pop to the schnoz is painful enough (and can create a dramatic flow of blood) to end the fight without too much damage inflicted on either party—which should be your ultimate goal.

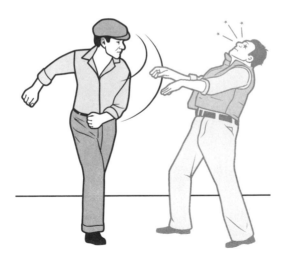

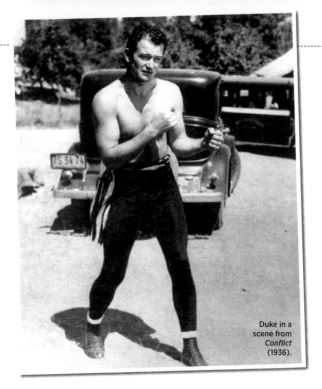

Duke in a scene from *Conflict* (1936).

HOW TO DEFEND YOURSELF IN A FIGHT

REAL MAN ALWAYS tries to avoid a fight, but if you can't then you better know what the hell you're doing to avoid serious injury. The tactics below should help you walk away from any brawl no worse for the wear.

1. *GET READY*
Assume a defensive position to minimize the harm you're about to receive, whether it's from fists or something worse.

Similar to the stance you assume when about to throw a punch (see page 200), you want to keep your chin angled down and bring your hands up to either side of your head while placing the opposite leg from your dominant hand in front of the other. If you're in the unlucky position of facing multiple assailants, try and get your back to a wall so you aren't taken unaware from behind.

2. *WATCH THE HANDS*

Your opponent usually won't strike you with his face, so keep an eye on his hands. This gives you more time to duck, dodge, block or counter punch when you see your assailant cocking his arm back to clock you one.

3. *GO FOR THE SOFT BITS*

Sure, it may be what some people call "fighting dirty" but you should think of it as "fighting for survival." Raking the eyes, hitting the "crown jewels," biting his ear Tyson-style...it's all fair game when you are in a fight for your life.

4. *ALWAYS MIND YOUR SURROUNDINGS*

Your arena of battle can often determine how serious the fight will get. If you are in a bar (drinking soda, of course) you need to be aware your opponent may grab a bottle as a weapon, escalating a regular rumble into a life-or-death struggle. Of course, you can always do the same, but that brings us to the last point....

5. *THE BETTER PART OF VALOR*

Don't fight. And if you have to fight, don't think of it in terms of "winning" but of "surviving." Look to stun or incapacitate, and then high tail it out of there. Every second you spend fighting is one where you risk permanent bodily harm, and even if you have the upper hand, do you really want a serious injury or death on your conscience (no matter how much the other guy may deserve it)? The answer is no.

HOW TO GIVE A GOOD HANDSHAKE

 HE HANDSHAKE WAS a greeting originally meant to show you weren't concealing a weapon and planning on murdering your new friend. Today we shake hands as a customary formal greeting as well as to casually test the mettle of the other person. Is she full of confidence? Does he enjoy the feel of crushing finger bones? These are questions the handshake answers. Make sure you pass your test with flying colors with the advice below.

1. *STAND AT ATTENTION*
Nothing sends a message of condescension like remaining seated during a handshake (the exception to this rule being if both of you are seated and it's not convenient for either of you to rise). Stand up, look the person in the eye and extend your hand. You should be aiming for the web between your thumb and index finger to make contact with the other person's to attain the proper grip.

2. *NICE AND FIRM*
The key to a good handshake is balance—too limp and it's like you're apologizing for your very existence, which is not a great impression to make. Too firm, and you'll leave the recipient wondering if you're about to sock him (or her) in the face. Giving a moderate squeeze should be enough to leave them impressed.

3. *PUMP IT UP*
While still looking the person in the eye, pump your hand up and down one to three times. The handshake shouldn't

last longer than five seconds, and even that is pushing it. Two or three seconds is more than enough.

4. *FRIENDLY FINISH*

When you let go of the other person's hand, maintain eye contact and continue your conversation so it's clear you're genuinely happy to meet him or her. Congratulations, you've just completed a great handshake!

NAVIGATING OTHER GREETINGS

There's more than one way to say "hello," beyond the tried-and-true handshake. Here's what to do when you find yourself in the company of people who aren't interested in grasping palms as a greeting.

1. If you're a man (which we assume), don't initiate a hug with a woman. In fact, you probably shouldn't go in for a hug with a man either. But if the other party initiates, accept it graciously, quickly and move on.

2. Certain people may say "hi" with a fancy-pants kiss on each cheek. Don't feel the need to kiss back, but (literally) turn the other cheek so they can finish their preferred greeting without you calling attention to the fact that it isn't your favorite way to say "howdy."

3. In Japan, you keep your arms straight to your sides and bend at the waist in a bow to say hello. Keep this bow at about 15 degrees, unless you are meeting the president, CEO of Toyota or someone of similar stature, in which case you want to dip down 30 degrees.

HOW TO PITCH A BASEBALL

ASEBALL IS AMERICA'S GAME, so being able to throw a decent pitch is almost a patriotic duty. You may not become a pro pitcher from studying a book, but the basics outlined below will at least give you a grasp on the fundamentals.

1. GET A GRIP

The first step in learning how to pitch is mastering the different ways to grip the baseball. Some of the most common are:

Two-seam Fastball: Grasp the baseball along the seams with your index and middle fingers while your thumb and your ring finger cradle the ball on its sides. A faster variant on this pitch is the four-seam fastball, which requires gripping the ball with your index and middle fingers so they are just slightly over the laces of the ball.

Curveball: Grasp the ball along the seams with your index and middle fingers, keeping them tightly together.

Changeup: Make an "OK" sign with your thumb and index finger and place it on the side of the ball, while your other fingers work to grasp the baseball.

Knuckleball: Grab the ball by the sides with your thumb and ring finger, digging your nails into the ball's cover and using your index and middle fingers to grasp the top of the ball. These two fingers should be bent so the knuckles are sticking out in the air.

2. STAND READY

Stand with your feet roughly shoulder-width apart with the ball in your dominant hand placed inside your glove (so the batter can't spot your grip and know what's coming down the

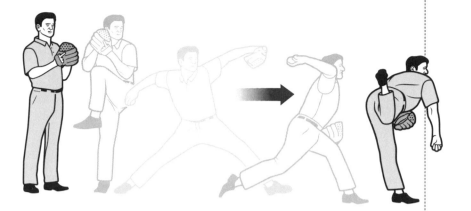

plate). Your body should be facing the catcher, with your toes pointed straight at him.

3. *WIND IT UP*

Take a small step back with your left foot (assuming you are right-handed—if you're not, do the opposite) and shift your weight to your left leg. Then pivot on the ball of your right foot so it is parallel to the catcher. Bring your left leg up until your thigh is parallel to the ground.

4. *BIG STRIDES*

Extend your left leg toward the catcher, taking a big step while your right (now back) foot kicks up to provide power— you can put speed on or off the ball by how aggressively you step and twist. At the same time, bring your arms downward with the back arm (the one with the hand holding the ball) dipping so it's nearly perpendicular with the ground. Now bring that arm in an upward arc toward the catcher, timing it so that arm is extended completely at the same time the left leg hits the ground.

5. *FOLLOW THROUGH*

Let the baseball fly from your grip—there shouldn't be any wrist action involved. Your arm should be extended as far as possible, and your back leg should be lifted up in the air from the momentum of your pitch.

HOW TO FLIRT WITH YOUR WIFE

O PARAPHRASE The Righteous Brothers (and *Top Gun*'s Maverick), it's easy to lose that loving feeling in even the strongest of relationships. But just because you've said "I do" doesn't mean you can't woo your lady in the way she deserves.

1. *EYES ON THE PRIZE*
The most basic principle underpinning all forms of flirting, from pulling Mary Jane's pigtails in fourth grade to exchanging bon mots over cocktails at a dinner party, is attention. Specifically, showering attention on her to make her feel as special as she is to you. Just because you put a ring on it doesn't mean these tried-and-true techniques should fall by the wayside. Make sure you aren't dividing your attention between your phone, the football game on TV and dinner, with her as a distant afterthought. Fully commit to the flirt.

2. *THE GENUINE ARTICLE*
While you want to go the extra mile to impress your wife and make her feel special, remember she fell in love with you—not some cheesy, bizarro version of yourself. Pay the missus the compliments and treat her the same way you did when you won her over, and don't try to become a completely different person. Unless...

3. *BACK TO THE BEGINNING*
...you think she'd be into that! While it may strike you as an exercise in corniess and awkwardness, many

couples spice things up by agreeing to go to a bar or restaurant separately and then "meeting" as pretend strangers. Role-playing like this may feel silly at first (and is definitely not for everyone), but nothing says "I love you" like remembering the first time your eyes locked across the room as your personal power ballad blasted on the jukebox, then repeating the line that swept her off her feet both then—and now.

4. SURPRISE HER IN PUBLIC

Most women (and men too) enjoy appropriate public displays of affection, so sending flowers to her work so her colleagues can see how much she is adored is a good call. Even something as simple and elegant as telling her you love her in front of your friends or holding her hand as you walk down the street is something that should send her heart aflutter.

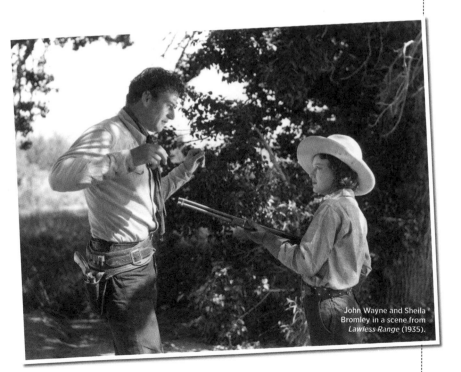

John Wayne and Sheila Bromley in a scene from *Lawless Range* (1935).

HOW TO DRIVE DEFENSIVELY

 ITTING THE OPEN ROAD is a lot of fun, but you should remember every time you get behind the wheel, you're taking control of a potentially lethal machine and need to comport yourself accordingly. Follow the below advice on defensive driving to make sure you head off trouble before it happens.

1. *DRIVE WITH YOUR HEAD*

Not literally, of course. Your brain is the most important organ you have when it comes to driving (and a lot of other things, for that matter). Handling a vehicle safely and defensively means making dozens of snap judgements that can mean the difference between a smooth ride and a disaster, so stay focused on the road. That means no music, no texting, no eating, no anything that distracts you from the task at hand.

2. *EXPECT THE WORST*

It would be nice if everyone else on the road always obeyed the traffic laws, in the same way it would be nice if your boss decided to double your salary and vacation time in appreciation for all the hard work you've done—in other words unlikely. Depend on the only person you can (hint: the same one that's reading this book right now). Instead of barrelling through the intersection just because you have the right of way, assume other drivers will run the red light or stop sign. This doesn't mean slow to a crawl through every green light, but definitely keep your eyes peeled for any reckless drivers.

3. *COUNT TO THREE*

No matter how diligent you are about checking your mirrors and keeping your eyes on the road, you can only react so quickly to a car that decides the middle of a four-lane expressway is an excellent spot to slam on the brakes. In ideal conditions (sun shining, birds singing, John Wayne movie waiting at home) you want to keep about three-seconds-worth of distance between you and the vehicle in front of you. When the person in front of you hits a landmark, count in your head how long it takes you to reach the same point to figure out your distance in terms of time. Of course, when driving through a hailstorm or any other dangerous conditions, you want to increase the distance to reflect the increased danger of a collision.

4. *STAY IN SIGHT*

Remember the goal of defensive driving is to minimize the risk of an accident, particularly with another driver on the road. But people can't avoid what they can't see, so don't spend a lot of time driving in the blind spot of that huge semi-truck on the highway. Also, be sure to signal all of your turns and lane changes to make sure there's no confusion about where you're headed.

HOW TO DRIVE A STICK SHIFT

HAT DO Steve McQueen's Mustang in *Bullitt* (1968), Sean Connery's Aston Martin in *Goldfinger* (1964) and your uncle's rusty '76 Pontiac Firebird Trans Am have in common? They all require you to know how to drive a stick shift in order to operate them. You may want to leave your uncle's junk heap in the garage, but do yourself a favor and study the information below to learn the basics of driving like a man.

1. *PRESS YOUR CLUTCH*

Before you start anything, press the clutch all the way down with your left foot. Just like an automatic vehicle, the brake and gas pedals are in the same place. But, on the far left you have an extra pedal called the clutch. Use your right foot for the gas and brake, but use your left foot to depress the clutch while you shift gears.

2. *ENGAGE THE PARKING BRAKE*

Never forget to set the parking brake while you're parked, or else your vehicle will roll. When you have the parking brake engaged, you don't have to depress the brake pedal, but you should always do so to stay safe.

3. *START IT UP*

Make sure your vehicle is in neutral, the middle position on your stick. Then, you can start your vehicle.

4. *KICK IT INTO GEAR*

Depress your clutch with your left foot and put your vehicle into first gear by moving the stick left and up. Release your parking brake, and rev up the engine to between 1,500 RPM and 2,000 RPM. If you rev it any

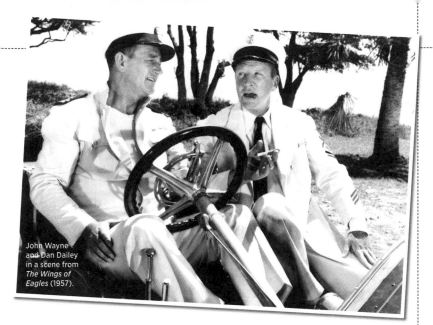

John Wayne and Dan Dailey in a scene from *The Wings of Eagles* (1957).

lower, your vehicle will stall, and you'll have to start 'er up again.

5. *RELEASE THE PRESSURE*

Slowly start lifting your left foot to ease off the clutch. Your vehicle should then start rolling slowly forward, and you should press the gas pedal slowly. When your engine reaches about 3,000 RPM, push your clutch down and move into second gear. When you need to stop, always push down your clutch and the brake, and move the gearshift back to neutral.

6. *KNOW WHAT GEAR TO BE IN*

Almost all vehicles have six gears. As said before, to move into first gear you move left and up. To change to second gear move left and down. Third gear is straight up, while fourth gear is straight down. Fifth gear is right and up, and sixth gear is right and down. You also need to switch gears according to your speed. When you're driving 0–15 mph, be in first gear. Everytime you go up another 10-15 mph, you should switch into the next gear. The same holds true for downshifting—when you slow down (or are driving down a hill) you should drop down a gear every 15 mph or so.

HOW TO PARALLEL PARK

ESSER DRIVERS may grow pale at the thought of having to parallel park, but just remember the instructions below and you'll find yourself cruising the streets at night looking for opportunities to show off your skills.

1. *SIGNAL AND ALIGN*

You're on a two-way street and have found a spot on the right side that you think you can most likely park in. It's time to turn on your signal and pull up three feet away from the car you want to park behind. Align your back tires with the other car's back bumper, so you're not crooked and sticking out into the street while parked.

2. *TURN TO THE RIGHT*

Put your vehicle in reverse and use your steering wheel to turn your wheels all the way to the right. Begin to slowly back up into the spot until you are at a 45-degree angle, then stop.

3. *A LITTLE TO THE LEFT*

After you stop, turn the wheels all the way to the left. Begin to slowly back up again until you're parallel with the curb. Make sure to keep straightening yourself out while parking.

4. *BE SAFE WHILE EXITING*

Open the door carefully. Make sure the road is clear to exit your vehicle. Cyclists are commonly found near parallel parking spots, so be cautious.

5. *WORK BACKWARDS*

If for some reason you're parking on the left side of the street (on a one-way, for example), use the preceding directions—just change left to right and right to left.

HOW TO FIND THE PERFECT PARKING SPOT

Grabbing the single parking spot in a crowded lot takes skill, patience and (most importantly) luck, but there are ways for maximizing your odds of victory.

1. Pick a row and commit to it, rather than driving around the whole lot in search of that space you feel is closer to the entrance of your destination. Don't fuss over the fact the row with an empty space is a little bit of a walk. On average, you are saving time and frustration by taking that space as opposed to driving back and forth.

2. If the lot is jam packed, find a place to wait for someone to leave rather than trying to find a new lot nearby. Odds are someone will leave eventually.

3. Be nice to the person who is vacating his or her parking space. Don't honk or yell or throw things. That's how you end up on the local news instead of in a parking space.

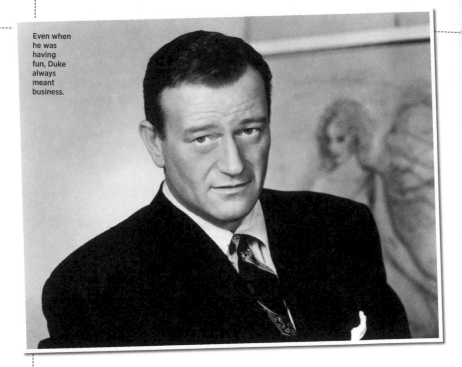

Even when he was having fun, Duke always meant business.

HOW TO PUT YOUR FOOT DOWN

A **NY GOOD RELATIONSHIP** lies on a solid foundation of compromise. You're never going to find someone with the same exact tastes as you (and probably shouldn't want to) so the secret to success—whether in a marriage, as a parent or a friend—lies in knowing which battles to pick. For the times you disagree and you absolutely have to insist on having your own way, there's still a way to let the other person know your feelings without things turning sour.

1. *PAY ATTENTION TO YOUR TONE*

Make sure your tone is positive and reassuring. "No" doesn't always require justification, and you've already made up your mind this time—there's no reason to be angry or forceful about it. Take the high road and be kind. Don't give attitude, but rather a smile and warm voice when talking through your reasons why.

2. *HONESTY IS THE BEST POLICY*

Always be honest. Do not beat around the bush. It could seem like you're creating excuses. Acknowledge the other person's wishes or wants, but make a clear direct statement as to why it's a no go. Don't leave it at that though. Try to lead into something positive.

3. *HEAR THEM OUT*

If they disagree with your assessment of the situation or feel hurt after kindly being turned down, hear them out. Concentrate and listen to what they have to say, but also be ready if things appear to be heading toward an argument. For kids, sometimes its easiest to end with a simple "Because I said so," but most children benefit from some explanation of reasoning beyond "I'm the boss and you're my unpaid employee until you're 18." For your peers or partner, there's no harm in letting them plead their case, but they should also know that eventually one of you has to give in—and it's not going to be you this time.

4. *GIVE AN ALTERNATIVE*

If you can, always have an alternative to your "no." For example, if something isn't fitting your schedule or you're just not in the mood, try and find another day to do it. If they want to engage in an activity that seems like it'd do at least one of you harm, offer up a safer but no less exciting option. If you're willing to meet halfway, you can even negotiate. In any situation, try to be considerate of why they want to do what they want to do. As long as you're clear about why you don't, they'll eventually get the idea.

HOW TO TALK TO A MECHANIC

OU MAY KNOW how to change your tires and your oil (see pages 138 and 142), but some car problems are best handled by the pros. When it comes time for you to talk shop, plenty of otherwise confident and in-command people find themselves bashful, intimidated by the sheer know-how possessed by a proper mechanic. Don't mumble and mutter to the guy (or gal) servicing your precious vehicle—speak with clarity and confidence by remembering the tips below.

1. *CLEAR COMMUNICATION*
You might not know what the exact issue is, but if you clearly explain what's going on with your vehicle, your mechanic will usually know what to do. When you start to see a problem, write down what you hear or see in order to accurately recall it for the pro. Don't withhold any information, or else they won't know what is truly going on with your vehicle. Think of your car as a body, and your mechanic as its doctor. You want to give them all the facts so they can make an accurate assessment, and recommend surgery if necessary.

2. *TAKE 'EM FOR A SPIN*
Some auto issues are better seen/heard/felt/smelled in person. That's why it's a good idea to take your mechanic out for a ride to fully show the problems you are facing with your vehicle. If your vehicle's

issue only happens in certain situations (driving uphill, idling in traffic, reversing over a curb) make sure to drive in those circumstances.

3. *GET EVERYTHING IN WRITING*
Discuss your issue, repairs and costs. Have everything itemized so you know exactly what you're paying for. Try to avoid negotiating costs, which are usually determined by the parts needed and the time it takes to make the repair. Once you have everything in order, get it all in writing for good measure. Nothing can be trusted just by word of mouth.

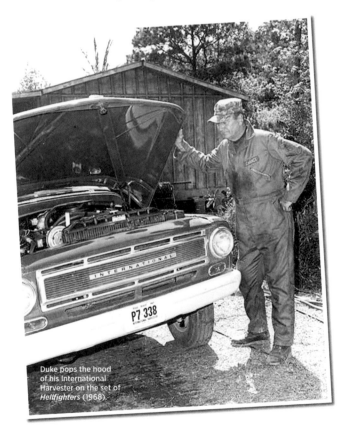

Duke pops the hood of his International Harvester on the set of *Hellfighters* (1968).

HOW TO MAKE A GOOD IMPRESSION

T'S OFTEN SAID that you only get one chance to make a first impression. That's why it's important to put your best foot forward, which means ensuring you don't look like a slob, smell like a dumpster and sound like a jackass. Read on to learn how to make sure the first impression you make is a lasting, positive one.

1. *LOOK THE PART*

A big part of making a good impression comes from feeling relaxed and confident in your own skin, but you don't want to be too comfortable. Even if you typically shower every third day and haven't had your hair combed since they checked for lice in elementary school, maybe take the time to spruce up your image. That doesn't mean becoming a completely different person and wearing a tuxedo when you're more of a T-shirt and sneakers kind of guy, but make sure you put on clean clothes and take care of basic hygiene.

2. *TAKE A HINT*

When carrying on a conversation, stick with innocuous topics but make sure they aren't so banal as to shut down the dialogue. "The weather is nice" is boring enough to draw a response of "Excuse me, but I believe I'm late for a root canal." On the other hand, "You wouldn't believe what I just did in that bathroom!" is not a great icebreaker. Try to comment on what's going on around you, ask about recent trips, their children or other topics devoid of land mines. Emily Post suggests never discussing politics or religion at parties, and the same goes for first chats with someone you've never met. If you're in doubt about what to discuss, perhaps share some of the other skills you've learned from this book. Nothing gets a conversation going faster than "Hey, did you know I can hot wire your car?"

3. *TO THINE OWN SELF BE TRUE*
In the end, the secret to making a good impression is to be yourself. Overanalyzing every question someone asks you and trying to contort yourself into the person you think he or she wants you to be will most likely lead you to acting like a weird robot whom nobody wants to spend time with. Relax, have fun and remember— they're probably just as nervous about meeting you as you are meeting them.

HOW TO IMPRESS YOUR BOSS

Among the most important people to impress is the one who signs your paychecks. Here are some tips for becoming employee of the month without also becoming a brownnoser.

1. Show up early. This is a bit of a no-brainer but is also a tough one for most workers. Of course, if your boss is worth impressing, he or she is looking for reliability in employees, and nothing says "I'm here to work" like literally being there.

2. Don't gripe to your boss. He or she really doesn't want to listen to complaints. Offering constructive comments on how to improve the work environment is fine, but just saying "Our office doesn't have windows and sucks" is not going to do you any favors.

3. Deliver as promised when it comes to work. Keep up your productivity and cement your reputation as someone on whom one can depend.

HOW TO WRITE A LETTER

G **ETTING A** handwritten letter in the mail from a friend or loved one seems to have gone the way of the gas lamp or horse-and-buggy, but the rarity of careful correspondence makes it that much more meaningful. Here's how to perfect a dying art.

1. *GET READY*
You probably didn't need to read this book to figure out you'll need a pen and some paper to write a letter, but don't think you can just grab some neon gel pen and a torn-out page of notebook paper. You should write in either black or blue ink, and the stationary you choose should have a nice heft to it. It's not uncommon for correspondence to be saved for years, so treat the material you choose with love and care.

2. *SEEK SOLACE IN SILENCE*
Writing a letter isn't brain surgery, but it does require a level of concentration and introspection that's become increasingly rare in the age of FaceTwitterGram. Find a quiet place free of clutter to write your letter in peace.

3. *GET INSPIRED*
Decades of writing emails has fooled most of the world into thinking that writing whatever pops into your head is the preferred way to communicate your ideas. But that's confusing convenience for what's right, something the rugged individualist never does. Think about if you really want to spend precious space telling the receiver of the letter what you had for breakfast this morning. Maybe you do! Just make sure you are writing with a purpose in every word you select.

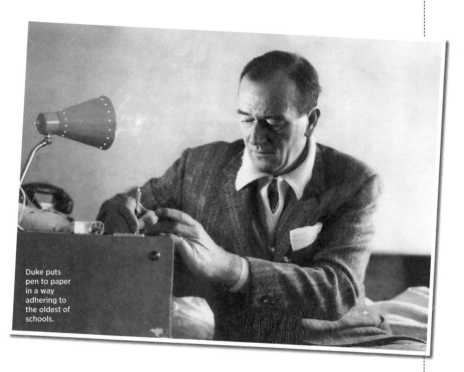

Duke puts pen to paper in a way adhering to the oldest of schools.

HOW TO IMPROVE YOUR HANDWRITING

Study these tips so your next missive doesn't resemble something scrawled out by a man who was raised by wild animals.

1. Make sure you are holding the writing utensil between the thumb and index finger, with the end of the pen or pencil resting on the web of your hand.

2. Pay attention to how much your letters are slanting on the page—too much makes the whole thing look sloppy.

3. Take every opportunity you get to write things out by hand. Grocery lists, quick notes, ideas for a John Wayne-themed party—practice makes perfect.

HOW TO KICK
A BAD HABIT

OBODY EVER SAW a cowboy on the psychiatrist's couch" is a quote often attributed to Duke, and there's certainly some truth in it: Some folks simply prefer to handle things on their own, and bad habits are no exception. For the rugged individualist, parting ways with a particular vice starts with recognizing you've gotten yourself caught up in one. In other words, self-improvement starts with self-awareness. What do I like about myself? What would I change if I could? With a little bit of grit and determination, you can kick whatever bad habits you may have to the curb to become an even better version of man you already are. So go on and read the tips below to get a handle on how to be a better you.

1. *BREAK IT DOWN*

One of the insidious ways our minds prevent us from working on eliminating our bad habits is by making them seem larger than life. Instead of focusing on "I want to quit smoking," which for many smokers seems like too ambitious of a change, think instead of how you want to smoke fewer cigarettes this week than last, with the goal of tapering off rather than quitting cold turkey. Slow and steady wins the race.

2. *GET IN TOUCH WITH YOUR FEELINGS*

Most of us have a predictable pattern of behavior that incorporates the bad habit, whether it's smoking or drinking or biting your fingernails. Trying to drop the habit without changing or addressing these behaviors is in some way an almost impossible task. For example, if you crush a six-pack every night to deal with anxiety, you may want to explore with a professional why you're such a jangle of nerves that it takes half a dozen drinks to calm you down.

3. *ASK FOR A SUB*
Constantly dwelling on the absence of the habit you used to enjoy (or at least compulsively partake in) is a sure-fire recipe for calling it quits on calling it quits. Instead, try to replace the unwanted action with a new, positive one. Spending too much time on your phone when you should be catching z's instead? Use that time to write in your journal about the day's events. Trying to cut back on the after-work booze? Turn happy hour into gym hour, or an hour of organizing your house or cooking dinner for you and your family. The possibilities are endless.

4. *TELL A FRIEND*
While the motivation for kicking the bad habit has to ultimately come from you, there's no reason you can't enlist the help of some friends by telling them you're trying to quit whatever it is you're trying to quit. The combination of peer pressure and a friendly ear to listen to your frustrations can sometimes be enough to see you through to your goal.

5. *STICK WITH IT*
Remember that depending on the habit, it can take a lot of attempts to kick it for good. Don't worry—nobody is keeping score and you shouldn't feel discouraged. Just try and identify what caused you to slip up, avoid that behavior, and try, try again.

HOW TO THANK A VETERAN

A S JOHN WAYNE would be the first to point out, freedom isn't free. And the heaviest price is usually paid by the men and women serving in our country's Armed Forces. The next time you want to pay your respects to a veteran but are unsure of how to properly express your appreciation, remember the following advice.

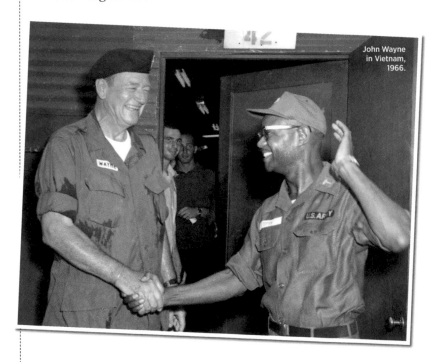

John Wayne in Vietnam, 1966.

1. *SOUND OUT*

This may come as a shock, but one of the best ways to thank a veteran for his or her service is to say "Thank you for your service" and leave it at that. Don't be flummoxed if the vet doesn't break down in tears by your gesture of gratitude—they tend to hear it a lot. That said, if the veteran is in the middle of proposing to a significant other or is dealing with a child's temper tantrum, maybe consider saving the "thank you" for another day.

2. *LISTEN UP*

As less and less of the country's population serves in the military, veterans risk becoming estranged from the vast majority of civilian society. If you have the time and a nearby, friendly veteran handy, take the time to ask about his or her experiences in the military. Common sense should be your guide. Open with something apolitical like "What do you miss most about your time in the service?" and let the veteran lead the conversation from there.

3. *MORE THAN WORDS*

You don't have to limit your appreciation to kind words. Volunteering through a local veterans organization can ensure your next Saturday is spent doing something more rewarding than watching reruns or falling asleep to golf.

HOW TO DANCE AT A WEDDING WITHOUT EMBARRASSING YOURSELF

 WEDDING should be a joyous occasion for the happy couple tying the knot, a day they'll remember for the rest of their lives. Don't be the guest who mars their happy memories with embarrassing dance moves that may or may not place a curse on the nuptials. Follow these basic tips to survive the dancefloor at the reception.

1. *CREATE COMMUNITY*

Unless you're overly confident, you never want to dance by yourself at a wedding. Whether it's with friends or your date, create a community to dance with just so you can have fun. Take them out on the dance floor and move to the music. Keep things simple.

2. *TOE TAP AND HEAD BOP*

No, this is not a cue to start tap dancing. Instead, listen to the music and tap to the beat. Eventually you'll either be stepping side to side, or back and forth. Just have your feet move to the beat. Nothing too drastic! That's always the first step to finding the beat for you to dance to. Then bop (nod) your head with it. This will allow your body to be in tune with the rhythm of the music.

3. *BOUNCE IT OUT*

Throw a little (the key word is little) bounce into your toe tapping. Don't be too stiff on the dance floor; you might just lose all your dance partners if you are. Put some bounce in your body and loosen up a little. Let the music guide you.

4. *IT'S ALL IN THE HIPS*

You have your feet tapping and head moving to the beat. Your body even has a little bounce. To take it to the next level, sway your hips. Your whole body should be moving at this point. You're here to celebrate and have fun, so why not look the part?

5. *SLOW DANCING? TAKE IT SLOW*

If you're slow dancing, ignore everything that was just stated. Take your partner's left hand in yours, put your right hand on her waist, hold her close and sway to the rhythm of the music.

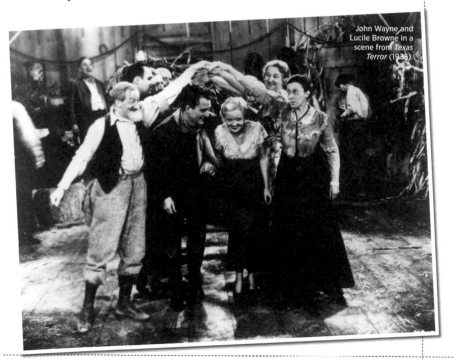

John Wayne and Lucile Browne in a scene from *Texas Terror* (1935).

HOW TO MAKE MOVING EASIER

ACKING UP AND MOVING to a new home is one of the most stressful experiences a person can suffer through. Even though relocating can herald a new beginning, it's still an old school pain in the ass. Learn how to make moving a little less rough by remembering the tips below.

1. *BAG YOUR HANGING CLOTHES*
Unhanging and packing all of the clothes in your closet is a major time waster. You can speed up the process by using garbage bags to pack them all directly into bunches without taking any of them off the hanger. Alternatively, many movers sell closet boxes, large refrigerator-sized boxes with a hanging bar inside, that essentially function as a mobile wardrobe. They cost a little more than trash bags, but will make you feel less like a vagrant ready to ride the rails with several bindles in tow.

2. *ORGANIZE YOUR WIRES*
Wires are some of the hardest things to pack and keep safe. Using an empty toilet paper roll can keep them all bunched up. After that pack that roll in a safe place (such as a small plastic bin or a bag you're carrying with you).

3. *SELL STUFF TO YOUR NEIGHBORS*
Moving is a good time to finally shed yourself of anything you've been hoarding. Having a yard sale to get rid of excess odds and ends will get you some extra space while also giving you some extra cash.

4. *COLOR CODE YOUR BOXES*

Assigning each room a color (e.g. "yellow for the kitchen") and then using that code to label your boxes will prevent you from mixing up your undies with your dish detergent, and will make unpacking a breeze. As you unload boxes from the truck or car, take them to their designated space and keep moving until all your boxes are unloaded.

5. *KEEP THE ESSENTIALS ACCESSIBLE*

There's nothing worse than needing an item of clothing, a toiletry or even a utensil when it's buried under a mountain of the trophies you were unable to unload at your pre-move yard sale. Try to create a small bag of the things you know you'll need before you unpack so that your arrival will be relatively stress free.

6. *MEET YOUR NEIGHBORS*

Now that you've arrived, get settled in and find time to introduce yourself to the folks who have been staring at you from their windows or the slats of their fence all day. A neighborhood is about community, and you'll want to foster one with the people you share property lines with. Otherwise you may find yourself packing up all over again.

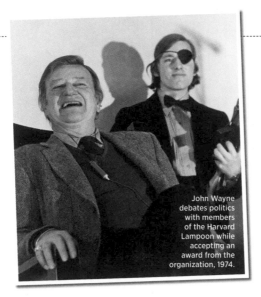

John Wayne debates politics with members of the Harvard Lampoon while accepting an award from the organization, 1974.

HOW TO HAVE A CIVIL POLITICAL DISCUSSION

UKE WAS A FRIEND to numerous presidents and politicians, but his loyalty was always to country over party. He wanted what was best for America and was never afraid to disagree with someone whose idea of progress was in conflict with what he felt was right. But just because you disagree with someone politically doesn't mean you need to get into a shouting match every time you get together. Read below on how to talk about the elephant (or donkey) in the room without having to cut ties with those you care about.

1. *ASSUME THE BEST*

Being genuinely interested in listening to another point of view means keeping an open mind, particularly about the other person's intentions. Treating the other person with respect goes a long way toward having a candid, fruitful exchange of ideas.

2. STUDY UP

It's tough to have a political discussion without a basic understanding of what you're talking about (though Lord knows plenty of people try), so give yourself a leg up on the average conversationalist by staying informed on the issues of the day. If the conversation starts to veer into territory you're unsure of, there's no shame in admitting you don't know much about the subject. Save the B.S. for the pasture.

3. USE PROPER NAMES

Modern political discourse has burdened us with plenty of nicknames and short-hand descriptions for every political viewpoint under the sun, and almost none of them are constructive. Leave the name-calling for the playground.

4. BE ORIGINAL AND OPEN

Anyone can repeat talk radio highlights or parrot the opinions presented on their preferred cable network. Part of the reason we engage with difficult dialogue is not just to change someone's mind, but to temper and hone our own beliefs. If all you're doing is repeating someone else's opinion you run the risk of lacking any of your own. If your opinions and beliefs seem in conflict with a well-reasoned argument, be open to the idea that you might, at least in this particular instance, be wrong. Think of the conversation as less of an argument and more of a discussion. You can't win a discussion. And you won't lose one either.

5. ALWAYS END WITH A HANDSHAKE

No matter how heated things get (and feel free to pull back from the conversation if they do) you should always endeavor to end your discussion with a handshake, hug or clap on the shoulder. It helps ensure there's no bad blood. After all, if you know you have to hug it out in the end, you're less likely to say something that'll make that hug harder.

HOW TO HAGGLE

NE OF THE SECRETS to living the life of a rugged individualist is refusing to take the world at face value. Refusing to take the easy path and forging your own way may mean you run into more difficulties than the average Joe, but it also leads you to more rewarding experiences, such as haggling for a good deal. Whether you're horse-trading for a new house or a square point shovel, learning to talk down the price isn't just a skill that saves you money. It can be fun.

1. *HAVE A HEAD FOR NUMBERS*
Specifically, you need to keep in mind two numbers when you enter any negotiation: the price you want to pay, and the highest price you are willing to pay. Ideally the number you end up at should land closer to the former than the latter, but haggling rarely works out that way. How do you determine the numbers that set your price range? Depending on what you're haggling over, finding the standard price could be as simple as a Google search or as complicated as having to ask other merchants who sell a similar product.

2. *QUIET, PLEASE*
It's not always possible, but you should always have the other party offer the first price. Otherwise, you run the risk of blurting out a starting price that may have been more than the merchant would have expected you to pay. Remember that as a buyer, you can only offer to pay more money, while the seller can only offer to charge you less (barring any external deals, which we'll get to later). Let the other party make the first move, and you may be pleasantly surprised by the initial offer.

3. *KEEP IT FRIENDLY*

Whatever your true feelings for the person on the other end of the haggle, it's going to be to your advantage to keep the conversation on the lighter side. That doesn't mean you can't drive a hard bargain, only that you shouldn't make the haggle feel as if it's a life-or-death, zero-sum negotiation. While both you and the other party most likely think your final decision will be the result of cold, hard logic, the truth is that charm plays a large part in pulling off a favorable haggle. That means if you act like a jerk, nobody is going to want to give you a good deal.

4. *BUT NOT TOO FRIENDLY*

Of course there's a difference between appearing friendly and desperate for a deal. If you exclaim "I need to have this!" then you only have yourself to blame when the other party calls your bluff when you try to nudge the price lower.

5. *GET CREATIVE*

Depending on the situation, everything is up for grabs during the haggle. If you can't get the price to within an acceptable range, start thinking of other ways you can add value to the deal, like asking the other party to throw in something else for free, or a discount on an item unrelated to the haggle at hand.

HOW TO SURVIVE A TRIP ABROAD

 MERICA IS the land of the free, home of the brave and all-around greatest country on the face of God's green Earth. But there's nothing wrong with taking a trip abroad to see the sights (and maybe more importantly, eat the food) of places both strange and exotic. When you do, you need to be careful—the rules you take for granted in the United States often don't hold overseas, and sometimes "tourist" can feel like another word for "target." Fear not (as if you would). Just keep in mind the following advice and bon voyage!

1. *GET SMART*

Or at least do the relevant research about what's going on in the individual countries you're going to visit. You don't need to know the main exports of the Philippines or the gross domestic product of Panama. However you should be aware if a city you'd like to visit is overrun by a drug cartel or if the Middle-Eastern area you're hoping to tool around is in the throes of an anti-Western revolt. One helpful resource is the State Department's online breakdown of travel warnings for Americans, found at *state.gov/travel*.

2. *KEEP YOUR VALUABLES CLOSE*

Depending on where you are planning to visit, you may stick out to the locals like a sore thumb. While the vast majority of people in any country aren't looking to harm or fleece you, conmen, pickpockets and worse do look at foreigners as targets of opportunity. Don't let essential documents such as your I.D. (especially the passport) out of your sight or off your person during the trip. Don't place them in your back pocket or in a backpack either, as they can easily be lifted from you by experts using sleight of hand. Wearing a money belt or a travel pouch under your shirt may feel a little inconvenient, but it's nothing compared to waiting in line for hours at the embassy trying to figure out a way to get back home.

3. *GET YOUR SHOTS*

While hopping over the border to Canada shouldn't require any additional vaccinations, some destinations have diseases and parasites not commonly found in the United States. Yellow Fever, rabies, Japanese encephalitis and hepatitis (A and B) are some examples of bugs you do not want to come down with that aren't typically covered by the vaccinations most Americans

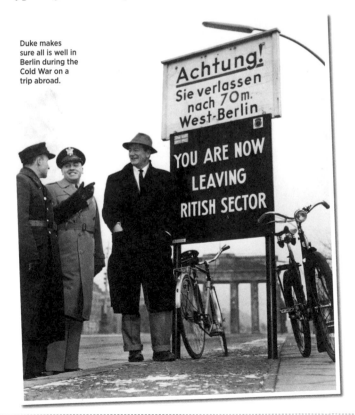

Duke makes sure all is well in Berlin during the Cold War on a trip abroad.

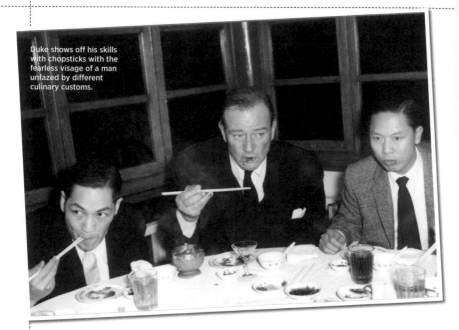

Duke shows off his skills with chopsticks with the fearless visage of a man unfazed by different culinary customs.

sign up for, so visit the Traveler's Health section of the website for the Centers for Disease Control and Prevention (CDC) at *cdc.gov/travel* to figure out which shots you might need before heading beyond our borders. Otherwise, you risk picking up a souvenir you could most definitely do without.

4. *HAVE FUN*

It's true you need to be careful when traveling abroad. But you need to balance that caution with the curiosity and sense of adventure that led you to venture beyond America's shores in the first place. You don't want to show off pictures of your trip only to discover you're looking at a slideshow of the interior of various McDonald's restaurants. Be friendly, try and talk with the locals and get out there and explore—with vigilance.

HOW TO SURVIVE A LONG PLANE RIDE (WITHOUT GOING CRAZY)

Back in John Wayne's day, flying was a much more luxurious experience for travelers, allowing people to start their vacations before they even arrived at their destinations (it was also much, much more expensive to fly, but we digress). Today it's more about a struggle to survive with your sanity intact, which the tips below should help you with.

1. Dress for comfort. You're going to be in a confined space for an extended period of time. Don't make things worse for yourself by showing up in a tuxedo or football pads or whatever. Loose-fitting, soft clothes will serve you well here.

2. Get up and stretch your legs every half hour. While sitting, keep your blood circulation up by occasionally lifting each foot, pointing your toes and tracing small circles. You can also do some knee lifts: raise your bent leg, contract the thigh muscles for 30 seconds, then relax and bring the leg back down.

3. If you are flying across multiple time zones, try eating and sleeping according to the time of your destination and not that of your departure. It may not make the flight itself more pleasant, but you'll thank yourself later when you have the leg-up on jet-lag.

HOW TO ASK FOR A RAISE

 OU MAY HARBOR a fantasy about moving out to the middle of the woods and living off the land, but chances are you're working for The Man (a person you should be trying to impress—see page 221). But that doesn't mean you have to be a sucker about it. Like John Wayne, you're a hard worker and a valuable asset to your boss, and you deserve to be rewarded for it. Make sure you get that raise by reading the tips below on how to ask for it like a boss.

1. *GATHER YOUR CASE*

Bosses don't typically dream of reasons to give their employees more money, so it's on you to build the case for why your take-home deserves a boost. Write down everything you've done that's contributed to the company's bottom line and demonstrates your value as a member of the team. Have you spent the last six years managing an account or project that's helped the company turn a profit? Talk to whomever you need to in order to ascertain how much. Remember, coming at your boss with hard numbers is always preferable than soft facts or feelings.

2. *SCHEDULE A MEETING*

Don't blurt out to your boss "I want more money!" the next time you happen to share the elevator with him or her. Nobody likes being caught by surprise. Instead, arrange to have some time set aside for the two of you to calmly and privately discuss the raise.

3. *SHOW RESPECT*

When presenting your case for the raise, you need to tread a fine line between confidence and arrogance. Be proud of your accomplishments and let your boss know you've made a difference for the company, but don't necessarily couch it in terms of "I did this, so gimme more money" (even if that's what you are essentially communicating). Instead, tell your boss you're happy to have been given the opportunity to shine, and additional compensation will ensure you will make even bigger contributions to the company's success.

4. *READ THE ROOM*

Did the company just lay off half the workforce or did your boss deliver a company-wide speech peppered with phrases such as "cutbacks" and "sacrifices?" Maybe now is not the time to ask for that raise. On the other hand, if they start putting ping-pong tables and new carpeting in the office, start building a case that details why you're as worthy of the company's investment as its new rec room.

HOW TO NEGOTIATE A HIGHER SALARY AT A NEW JOB

Getting a job offer should always bring a smile to your face, but more importantly it should add greenbacks to your wallet. Don't be a sucker and leave money on the table just because you were too bashful to ask for it.

1. Do your research on what the new job should pay, taking into account where you are working and how much experience you bring to the table. Websites such as *payscale.com* or *glassdoor.com* can help you get started, but don't be afraid to ask people you trust in your field for additional info.

2. If possible, enter negotiations over the phone. If you can swing it so you talk about it in person, even better.

3. When email is your only way of negotiating, make sure you are both respectful and clear about the reasons you think you deserve a higher salary. How you act now can set the tone for your career.

HOW TO THROW A TASTEFUL BACHELOR PARTY

HE TRADITION of the stag night before the wedding is a long and somewhat-seedy one, but a bachelor party doesn't have to involve scantily clad women and shots of tequila. What's important is that your friend has a night (or weekend) of camaraderie to celebrate a life milestone. Read the tips below to ensure you send him off in style and not in shame.

1. *ASSEMBLE YOUR CREW*

The appropriate size and scope of the bachelor party will vary according to individual. A general rule of thumb is that you shouldn't invite so many people that you can't reasonably coordinate everyone's schedules, but it shouldn't be so small that you could all fit into a compact car. This is about the groom-to-be, so you should invite people from across different friend groups so long as they are close to the main man. Generally speaking, all groomsmen should be invited, unless the groom has only named someone a groomsman out of obligation (future brother-in-laws or the bride's best male friend who still isn't over her are classic examples). Above all, make sure there's no beef between any of the men on the trip—you don't want any arguments (or fist fights) to sully the good time.

2. *TIMING IS EVERYTHING*

Just as a matter of common sense, don't schedule the festivities the night before the wedding. For that matter, the weeks before the nuptials usually demand a lot of planning and attention from the couple, so you're probably better off scheduling the bachelor party at least one month before the big day. If people need to travel from points afar, make sure you invite everyone and send them the details well in advance of the party (say three months) so they have time to clear their schedules.

3. *GET CREATIVE*

Sure, a night of (legal) debauchery may provide great material for a lifetime of embarrassing stories, but why not arrange for something more memorable and, more importantly, respectful to the bride-to-be. A weekend hiking in the woods, whitewater rafting or a poker night with John Wayne movies can provide a great bonding experience minus the vice.

4. *SHARE THE BURDEN*

Whatever the costs of the entertainment, it's fair to split the bill evenly between everyone invited (minus the man of the hour), but make sure the crew agrees on that first before springing a bill on them at the end of the celebration. If the party takes place out of town for the groom, don't feel the need to foot his airfare or hotel room, but the only time he should reach for his wallet during the trip itself is when he shows the bouncer his I.D.

HOW TO APOLOGIZE

"NEVER APOLOGIZE, MISTER.** It's a sign of weakness" is a great line Duke as Capt. Nathan Brittles delivers in *She Wore a Yellow Ribbon* (1949). But in the real world, we sometimes fall short of John Wayne's high standards and have to express regrets for our blunders. A true apology should be well articulated and filled with a real promise that the mistake will never happen again—one of which even Duke could be proud.

1. *SAY YOU'RE SORRY*

It's only a first step but it's a very important one. So many people just stop at this and figure the problem is

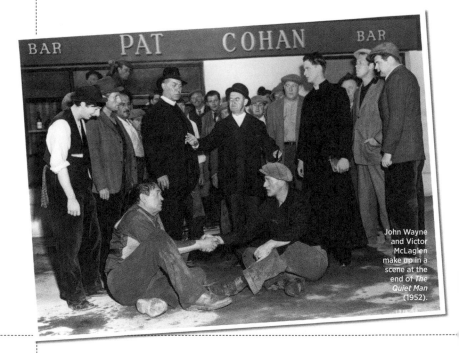

John Wayne and Victor McLaglen make up in a scene at the end of *The Quiet Man* (1952).

solved, and that's a very careless mistake. Don't just say "I'm sorry," say "I apologize" or "I'm sorry for…" to show that you really are about to mean what you're going to say next.

2. ARTICULATE WHY YOU'RE GUILTY

Now it's time for the hard part. While it can be difficult to truly dig into what you did wrong, you have to come clean if you want that person to truly forgive you. Get specific about why what you did was wrong, and about how it hurt the person you affected. Don't skimp out on the details, it may be difficult but this is an important step in showing you've internalized your guilt.

3. MAKE A DEDICATION FOR THE FUTURE

Now explain how you're not going to do this again going forward. Explain what life changes you're going to make that will prevent you from making these same mistakes. Once again, be specific. It will show you really do mean you'll follow the plan you've laid out.

4. ASK FOR FORGIVENESS

So many people just expect forgiveness. But absolution should never be expected, it has to be earned. Asking for forgiveness will show that you really have been humbled by your mistakes and that you sincerely hope to change. A sincere plea for forgiveness is typically all a wronged party wants to hear and will help bandage any damage you've caused. And remember, "I'm sorry you feel that way" isn't an apology, it's a cop out.

HOW TO HANDLE A MINOR TRAFFIC ACCIDENT

 T HAPPENS to us all. While you can't just leave once you're in a minor traffic accident, knowing the correct thing to do will minimize the amount of time you spend there.

1. *CONFIRM EVERYONE'S SAFE AND PARK YOUR CAR*
Once you've ensured everyone's OK, get your car into a safe place. Try to get yourself to the side of the road to avoid any oncoming traffic. You might be disoriented from the accident so don't forget to put your vehicle in park and then turn it off. Get out of your car and evaluate the situation, being sure to cordon off your car with traffic cones, flares or at the very least, turn on your hazard lights.

2. *CALL FOR ASSISTANCE*
Call the police, even in the most minor of accidents. A police report will usually provide objective details on the event, which will be invaluable when it comes to processing an insurance claim. While explaining the event to a police officer, be careful not to admit blame or to place too much blame on the opposing party, as it won't help your case. If anyone is injured, even if it seems minor, make that known during your 911 call as well.

3. *KEEP USING YOUR HEAD*

In order to file an insurance claim you need a fair amount of concrete info. Make sure to note the driver and passenger names, vehicle descriptions, contact and insurance info of parties involved, the location of the accident, license plate numbers and the names and badge numbers of the police officers on the scene.

4. *FILE A CLAIM*

If you're up to it you can use the information you've acquired to make an insurance claim, so do it right away. Use the internet or call your insurance provider. Since you always keep a copy of your insurance details in your wallet or glove box, you'll know you have them on hand to get a head start on filing. What's that? You don't keep your insurance info handy in your car? Fix that, pilgrim.

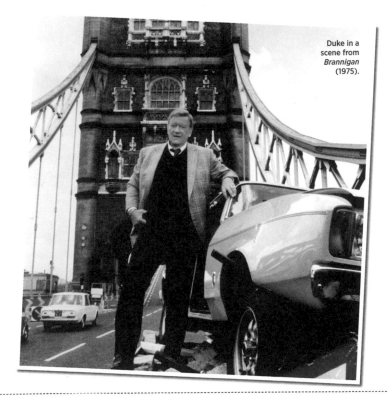

Duke in a scene from *Brannigan* (1975).

HOW TO WIN AT POKER

HESS MAY BE the game of kings (and of at least one Duke, given how much John Wayne loved it) but poker is the name of the game for any red-blooded American ready to win his fortune via a dance with Lady Luck. But as any player worth his (or her) salt will tell you, there's a good deal of strategy involved— too much for us to impart on these pages. However, the tips below should set you on the path to taking home more money than you brought to the table—most of the time.

1. *DON'T BET YOUR RENT MONEY*

The first rule of winning poker is to make sure losing the game won't have disastrous consequences for you. Don't bet actual money your life depends on, such as the cash set aside for the heating bill or groceries. Sure, there's a certain thrill of playing with the knowledge that you're just a bad hand away from crashing on your buddy's couch next month but...you still would have to crash on your buddy's couch. It's not worth the risk.

2. *BET WITH YOUR BRAIN*

One of the most common mistakes beginners make at the poker table is undermining their own good fortune with a poor betting strategy. If you find yourself holding a royal flush, pushing in your whole pile of chips will most likely signal to the other players that they should fold. Congrats! You've just blown a great hand on a meager pot that won't even pay for gas money home.

3. *DON'T FEAR THE FOLD*

Obviously you can't do this for every hand, but novice players have a seemingly pathological aversion to folding. The truth is, most hands you'll draw in poker aren't going to be great. Sometimes you can bluff your way to victory, but more often than not you need to cut your losses and save your money for the right hand.

4. BE A QUICK STUDY

One aspect of the game you should always be studying is how your opponents' betting matches with the cards they have. If you can determine their patterns and behaviors, you can (somewhat) predict the strength of their hands based on their bets alone. For example, if someone makes big bets and it's consistently revealed he or she does so only when they have a good, winning hand, you might not want to take that "all-in" seriously.

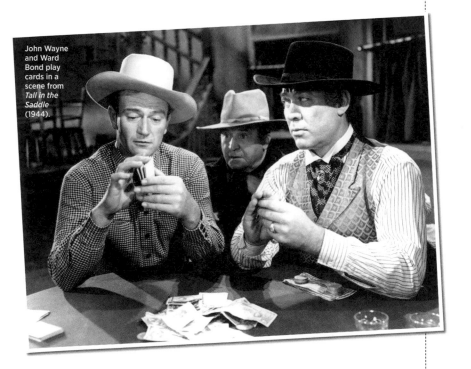

John Wayne and Ward Bond play cards in a scene from *Tall in the Saddle* (1944).

HOW TO SURVIVE A NIGHT OF KARAOKE

HILE WE ARE SORELY tempted to simply write "Don't go" as the instructions for this skill, there are times that, despite your best efforts, you get dragged to the ultimate chamber of horrors—the karaoke bar. Reverberating with the shrieking laughter of 20-something girls as their friend sings off-key to Beyonce and the jingle-jangle of tambourines trying to keep beat to Meat Loaf, these establishments can break lesser men. But not you.

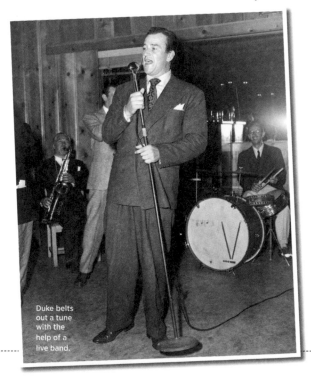

Duke belts out a tune with the help of a live band.

1. *KNOW YOUR LIMITS*

If you have the vocal range of Whitney Houston or Prince, then go ahead and queue up "I Will Always Love You" or "Purple Rain." But because you're reading an entry titled "How to Survive a Night of Karaoke," it's safe to assume your vocal abilities are more... modest. Use common sense and try and stick with songs that don't require 10 key changes or for you to hit ear-splitting high notes. Hint: Artists such as Bruce Springsteen or George Strait can be your friends here, as they generally stay in a range most people can mimic. Alternatively, take a late-era Rat Pack approach to your tunes and just rhythmically talk your way through the stuff you don't feel like singing.

2. *MOUNT THE HORSE*

Delivering a spirited but off-key rendition of "Don't Stop Believin'" isn't the worst thing you can do—though it's pretty close. What you should truly dread is half-mumbling your way through a song, inflicting three to four minutes of extreme awkwardness on the audience thanks to your cowardice. If you can't hit the notes, at least give people a show—twirl the mike, sing loudly and generally go big. With karaoke, it's better to go out with a bang than a whimper.

3. *DOUBLE DUTY*

If it looks like you're about to be corralled for some time on the mic, try and pick a duet so you can rope someone else in on sharing singing duties with you. Two heads (and in this case sets of vocal cords) are better than one.

HOW TO SHOOT POOL

 OOL IS NOT a game you can fake your way through with brute force. You need to have a precise and focused mood to ensure every ball goes where you want it to. Nerves or aggressiveness will only hamper your shot, and there's nothing more nerve wracking than being out of your depth. Follow these very precise steps to ensure you don't get hustled (or beat by your 11 year-old nephew).

1. PROPERLY POSITION YOUR HANDS ON THE POOL CUE

Hold the back end of the cue with your dominant hand. Make sure to grip it about one inch behind where the cue is evenly balanced. With your nondominant hand, make a circle around the front of the cue using your thumb and index finger. Rest the cue on your middle finger and spread out your pinky and ring finger to give it support.

2. STAND DOWN

Place the foot on the same side as your nondominant hand in the front with the other foot two feet behind you. Lean onto the table and make sure the cue is directly below your chin. Support yourself with your front foot, but allow for the flow of your body's momentum to go from your back foot forward.

3. PREPARE FOR THE SHOT

Get a good eye on the ball so you see directly where you plan to shoot and where it will go. Keep your cue positioned parallel to the table so it doesn't shoot wildly. You want to imagine a line from your stick through the cue ball and into the ball you're intending for it to strike.

4. *SHOOT*

Rather than going for a quick, powerful shot you want to go for more of a smooth and precise motion. Accelerate your speed as the cue approaches the ball so that the longer shot will do a better job of pushing the ball. Keep your eye on the target ball through your cue's impact with the cue ball. Make sure to fully follow through with your shot, so that it's a relaxed motion without any jumpy movements. This will ensure that the stick travels straight. And if your stick travels straight, there's a pretty good chance the ball will too.

5. *KNOW THE ANGLES*

You'll rarely get an opportunity where the cue ball lines up with your target ball and the pocket, so it is important you know how to bank the ball off the sides of the table (called the rails) or "cut" a ball by hitting it or grazing it on its sides in order to sink shots. A ball hitting the rail at one angle will always bounce off at the same angle, so try to picture in your mind the path of the ball hitting the rails based on this mathematical axiom. Finally, math class pays off!

6. *DON'T FEAR THE BRIDGE*

There's no shame in admitting your arms just aren't long enough for a shot in the middle of the table. After all, not everyone is built like Duke. It's better to use a bridge to extend your reach than to lose a game with your vanity.

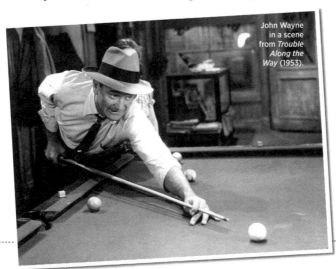

John Wayne in a scene from *Trouble Along the Way* (1953).

HOW TO PROPERLY FOLD AN AMERICAN FLAG

D UKE WAS NEVER SHY about his patriotism, and chances are if you're reading this book you also fly Old Glory outside your home. Which means you probably know the symbol of the greatest nation on Earth shouldn't be left hanging outside like a dirty bed-sheet at night (or in inclement weather). There's a definite, time-honored tradition to properly stowing the flag, which—if you don't know—you'll know now.

1. *DOWN TO UP*
First, take the flag and lay it perfectly flat on a table. Fold it in half evenly from the bottom up, so the striped section completely covers the Union (the blue field with fifty stars).

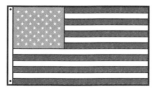

2. *ONCE MORE WITH FEELING*
Take the bottom edge and fold it to the top edge once more—now

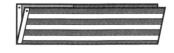

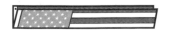

the Union as well as the stripes should be showing. Be sure to keep the creases tight and that the corners align.

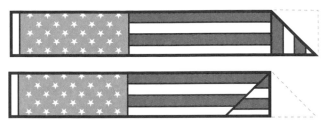

3. *KNOW ALL THE ANGLES*

Take the top-right corner of the striped edge, and fold it diagonally down so it meets the bottom edge. You've just created a triangle. Take the bottom-right corner of that triangle and fold it to the left, parallel to the bottom edge. You've made another triangle, which you'll use to take you into the big finale.

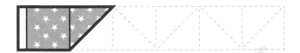

4. *KEEP IT COMING*

Now keep folding this triangle toward the left until the entire flag ends up as a triangle. Typically, that means two more folds parallel to the bottom edge, two parallel to the top edge and two more parallel to the bottom edge.

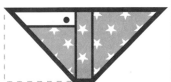

5. *TUCK IT IN*

Create a new triangle to tuck the remainder of the flag into the pocket created by Step 4, and congratulate yourself on your respectful display of patriotism.

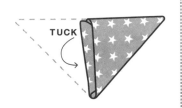

TUCK

Media Lab Books
For inquiries, call 646-838-6637

Copyright 2018 Topix Media Lab

Published by Topix Media Lab
14 Wall Street, Suite 4B
New York, NY 10005

Printed in China

ISBN-13: 978-0-9993598-8-4
ISBN-10: 0-9993598-8-6

CEO Tony Romando

Vice President and Publisher Phil Sexton
Senior Vice President of Sales and New Markets Tom Mifsud
Vice President of Brand Marketing Joy Bomba
Vice President of Retail Sales & Logistics Linda Greenblatt
Director of Finance Vandana Patel
Manufacturing Director Nancy Puskuldjian
Financial Analyst Matthew Quinn
Brand Marketing Assistant Taylor Hamilton

Editor-in-Chief Jeff Ashworth
Creative Director Steven Charny
Photo Director Dave Weiss
Managing Editor Courtney Kerrigan
Senior Editor Tim Baker

Content Editor James Ellis
Content Designer Michelle Lock
Art Director Susan Dazzo
Associate Art Director Rebecca Stone
Assistant Managing Editor Holland Baker
Designer Danielle Santucci
Associate Photo Editor Catherine Armanasco
Assistant Photo Editor Stephanie Jones
Assistant Editors Alicia Kort, Kaytie Norman
Editorial Assistants Courtney Henderson-Adams, Sean Romano

Co-Founders Bob Lee, Tony Romando

Photo Credits: p8 Keystone/Getty Images; p12 AF Archive/Alamy; p37 Photo 12/Alamy; p47 Everett Collection; p68 Everett Collection;
p79 INTERFOTO/Alamy; p98 AF Archive/Alamy; p132 Everett Collection; p155 Bettmann/Getty Images; p175 AP Images; p191 Everett
Collection; p194 Keystone Pictures USA/Alamy; p197 Everett Collection Historical/Alamy; p213 Everett Collection; p216 John Springer
Collection/Getty Images; p232 PL Gould/IMAGES/Getty Images; p247 Pictorial Press/Alamy; p253 Everett Collection

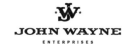